Dedicated to
The Two Percent Club.
Thank you. For everything.

Other works by Jo Kline, J.D.
(also written under the pseudonym Jo Kline Cebuhar, J.D.)

Multistate and Iowa
Health Care Advance Directive forms

**The practical guide to
Health Care Advance Directives**

EXIT – A novel about dying

SO GROWS THE TREE
Creating an Ethical Will
The legacy of your beliefs and values,
life lessons and hopes for the future

**The Workshop Edition of
SO GROWS THE TREE**

Whose big idea was that?
Lessons in giving from the
pioneers of value-inspired philanthropy

Last things first, just in case...
The practical guide to Living Wills
and Durable Powers of Attorney for Health Care

Principles of Tax-deferred Exchanging
(1996 and 2001 editions)

TABLE OF CONTENTS

CHAPTER ONE

Why I wrote this book.
Why you should read this book.

It all started with the Hula-Hoop.

Twenty-five million twirling whirling plastic rings were sold in 1958—in four months.[1] What causes a retail phenomenon of those proportions? Oddly enough, it's the same thing that prompted me to write this book about health literacy: the ubiquitous Baby Boomers born between 1946 and 1964. Today, 75.4 million Boomers are the moving force behind a perfect storm that's peeking over the horizon. It is the inevitable clash of: 1) this cohort of aging Americans; 2) the dwindling financial and human resources available to address their needs; and 3) our pervasive lack of health literacy.

The number of Americans aged 65 and older will increase by 60 percent over the next 13 years. And they just keep on coming: By 2050, those 65 and older will have doubled in number, while the group of Americans aged 85 and older will have tripled in size.[2] And there's no question that when it comes to medical emergencies, chronic conditions and caregiving demands, the Boomers are high maintenance folks.

At the end of the postwar baby boom, nearly 40 percent of Americans were 18 years of age or younger.[3] For over 65 years, Boomers have had a major influence on every segment of the American consumer economy from baby food to pension fund viability. Their most recent impact? The imploding Medicare budget, coupled with the rising shortage of health care workers caused by the retirement of—you guessed it—the Boomers. Simply put, if you've visited a long-term care facility recently, reimagine it with twice as many residents and half as many employees. Yikes.

That brings us to the third and final component of this perfect storm, a lack of health literacy. In 2006, I wrote a book on Advance Care Planning, *Last things first, just in case,* that focused on having a Living Will and a Durable Power of Attorney for Health Care in anticipation of end-of-life decision making. While preparing to write an updated edition of that book in 2014, I thought back on what readers and audience members have shared with me for nearly a decade. There is a common theme to the stories of their long and winding journeys with sick and dying loved ones: *"If only we'd understood, we would have made different choices."* I finally got it. For over forty years, legal and medical professionals have been harping about the importance of preparing for decision making that may be necessary during the final days or weeks of life. It turns out they were wrong—and when I say "they," I mean me, too.

Health care has become increasingly complex over the past few decades, in both its methodology and the decision making it requires. Rather than choosing whether to use life prolonging measures for a loved one close to death, today's decision maker is much more likely to be managing the long-term treatment of multiple chronic conditions. Navigating the system as patients and as caregivers, we face countless care options as illnesses progress over years or even decades. As those who share their stories with me already know, only in hindsight are we able to recognize that a decision made hastily or without sufficient information can have far-reaching and unintended consequences.

As you would expect, the perfect storm impacting society at large translates into tangible and critical challenges for individuals—that's you and me and those we care for and about. Reduced reimbursement rates force doctors to opt out of Medicare. Fewer providers means longer wait times. And exactly who is going to answer your hospital call button in 2024 when there are over one million unfilled nursing jobs?[4] Is there a way to preserve the rights to informed consent and patient autonomy amid this catastrophic collision of supply and demand?

We can't change demographics. As for reversing the lack of resources, it won't be accomplished overnight—if at all—and definitely not before the next medical crisis is at hand for one of us or someone we care for. That leaves one element of this inevitable storm in our control as individuals: health literacy.

A study done by the U.S. Department of Health and Human Services concluded that over one third of American adults have basic or below basic health literacy skills. In practical terms, less than half of American adults understand their prescription labels and only one in five knows how to interpret disease symptoms. That's far less than what's needed to fully function in today's complex health care system.[5] Thousands more studies have been done to measure whether a lack of health literacy affects health care. Not surprising, people with lower health literacy are hospitalized more, have less preventive care, are more likely to misuse prescriptions and have a higher mortality rate,[6] further evidence of the need for sharpened decision making skills in a health care system that is unprepared for the tsunami heading its way.

Recommendations for how providers can improve physician-patient communication have come from those studies, and many are just plain disturbing: speak like you're talking to your grandmother; avoid medical terms; use only one- or two-syllable words; and don't provide too much information.[7] Simply put (so even you and I can understand), the suggested remedy for patients' lack of health literacy is for health care professionals to seriously dumb down their messaging.

I disagree. What's more, I have a better idea.

As the patient in the patient-provider relationship, only *you* can preserve your right to informed consent and autonomy by taking the steps necessary to achieve health literacy and be a skilled and effective decision maker. Only *you* can prepare your trusted loved ones to act as informed substitute decision makers, if the need ever arises. As importantly, only *you* can achieve the health literacy needed to do the best job possible as an advocate for someone else.

Yes, it was a lightbulb moment for me.

Preserving the right to informed consent and to receive competent and compassionate health care and end-of-life care is entirely dependent on the decision maker's ongoing level of health literacy.

Literacy of any kind is the ability to proficiently read, write and speak a language and health literacy is no exception. It means recognizing when, how and where to access, process and understand basic health information and services needed to make informed decisions concerning medical treatment and care. Since the 1970s, medical decision making has focused on life's end, through the process of Advance Care Planning. No question, Advance Care Planning goes hand-in-hand with health literacy, but the implications of health literacy extend far beyond preferences for the use of life prolonging measures. Health literacy includes the tools and resources needed to make informed decisions regarding preventive, routine, emergency and, of course, end-of-life care:

- Selecting appropriate health insurance, providers and services.
- Knowing the preventive tests and procedures to undergo as we age.
- Properly preparing for a diagnostic test and understanding the results.
- Evaluating symptoms and knowing what medical care to seek.
- Responding properly in an emergency.
- Interpreting probabilities concerning disease, therapies and side effects.
- Managing a chronic medical condition.
- Having the knowledge and skills to properly use medical devices.
- Exploring available options for post-operative care and rehabilitation.
- Being a fully-informed user of prescribed and over-the-counter medications.
- Assessing pain and seeking pain relief alternatives.

- Knowing the rights and responsibilities of a health care advocate and proxy.
- Choosing the most qualified persons to act as health care advocate and proxy.
- Maintaining a healthy lifestyle.

To illustrate the difference between being educated and achieving health literacy, imagine a brain surgeon learns he has stage IV pancreatic cancer. Like most of us, he hears only white noise after the word *cancer* and has no idea what to do next. Wait— are we saying a medical expert on the workings of the human brain can lack health literacy? Absolutely, if he isn't already familiar with the lingo or treatment options for pancreatic cancer *and* he doesn't have a process in place to access what he needs to make informed decisions for himself.

Throw in that the brain surgeon doesn't speak English. We can overcome the language barrier with a translator, but the brain surgeon still lacks health literacy if he doesn't know what questions to ask and isn't able to calmly evaluate his treatment options—two of health literacy's core elements. You see, without a process at the ready for medical decision making, even the smartest person in a room full of really smart people can lack health literacy.

Although it is not the goal of health literacy to make you an expert on specific health care topics, there are some essential concepts to master, such as appreciating the right to informed consent and not signing anything until you understand it. In general, though, health literacy is having the tools you need to find the answers you need to exercise your rights as a fully informed patient.

This guy falls into a hole . . .

Walking down the street, just minding his own business, this guy falls into a deep, steep hole. There's no way he can get out on his own. Then a doctor passes by and the man shouts up, "Hey doc, can you help me out?" The doctor scribbles a prescription, throws it down the hole and moves on. Along comes a priest and the man yells, "Father, I'm stuck in this hole. Can you give me a hand?" The priest writes a prayer on a slip of paper, tosses it into the hole and keeps walking.

Then a friend walks by. Up from the hole comes, "Hey, buddy, it's me! Help me out, will ya?" The friend jumps in the hole. The man turns and looks at him, astonished, "What are you doing? Now we're both stuck here."

The friend smiles at the man and says, "Yeah, but I've been down here before and I know the way out." [8]

I have a confession to make. I'm no health care expert. Although I'm an attorney, mostly I'm someone who has traveled her own journey in the health care system and alongside others, and with each new experience, realized how little I knew. That's what prompted me to learn everything I could about medical decision making and end-of-life care. So, first and foremost, I'm a patient, just like you, except that I've already discovered the tools needed to achieve and practice health literacy.

This book is intended for anyone involved in the process of medical decision making. Yes, I focus on the patient's perspective, but everything that applies to a patient applies equally to anyone acting on behalf of a patient who no longer has decision making capacity, whether as the patient's proxy or provider.

Before we go any further, I make two promises to you, the reader:

• First, I don't agree that the way to overcome the lack of health literacy is to dumb down patient-provider communication. I think you're plenty smart, you just haven't been given the tools you need to get the information you need—until now. I will not patronize you.

• Second, because you are reading this book, I know you are serious about being an empowered medical decision maker for yourself or as the health care advocate for someone else. I am committed to help you accomplish that goal.

CHAPTER TWO

℘)⟨℞

Informed decision making and patient autonomy

The legal story of informed medical decision making begins with a parent's worst nightmare: the 2:00 a.m. phone call. On April 15, 1975, an unconscious 21-year-old Karen Ann Quinlan was transported to a hospital in Newton, New Jersey. She remained in a vegetative state, what we would call irreversible unconsciousness. Whether her father had the right to honor Karen Ann's wishes and remove her ventilator was ultimately decided by the New Jersey Supreme Court in 1976.[9]

In the Matter of Karen Ann Quinlan was a landmark case for several reasons:

•   For most Americans, it was their first exposure to the bioethics raised by Karen Ann's medical condition: the question of whether to withdraw life support.

•   As we came to understand the vegetative state, we realized that modern medicine is now capable of prolonging life indefinitely in many cases.

•   The New Jersey Supreme Court's ruling that Karen Ann's father could remove her ventilator began a shift from the paternalistic care model to the acknowledgement of a patient's right to informed consent and autonomy.

In 1983, seven years after the *Quinlan* decision, 25-year-old Nancy Beth Cruzan was thrown from her car in an accident that left her in cardiopulmonary arrest; she never regained consciousness after resuscitation. Four years later Nancy Beth's family asked to remove the feeding tube prolonging her life, a request that was denied by the state-owned hospital caring for her. In *Cruzan v. Director, Missouri Department of Health (1990),* the U.S. Supreme Court made it clear there is no legal presumption that favors the removal of life prolonging measures, so Missouri could require clear and convincing evidence of the patient's preference for that choice. Once it was shown that Nancy Beth had said *"she would not wish to continue her life if sick or injured unless she could live at least halfway normally . . .,"* the feeding tube was removed. Nancy Beth Cruzan passed away in 1990.[10]

These court cases confirmed that a patient's right to privacy and due process compel health care providers to obtain *informed consent* from a patient prior to any treatment, with very narrow exceptions, such as an emergency. Informed consent means voluntarily agreeing to, refusing to agree to or requesting the withdrawal of a medical procedure. (Note that there is no difference under the law or medical ethics between *withholding* treatment and *withdrawing* a medical procedure that has already been started, including life prolonging measures.)

Truly informed consent can be given only after a full understanding of the foreseeable risks, benefits, possible alternatives, uncertainties and the option of having no treatment. *Quinlan* and *Cruzan* made it clear that the right to informed consent does not vanish if the patient lacks decision making capacity on a temporary or permanent basis. That simply means a patient-appointed health care proxy, a court-appointed guardian or a surrogate decision maker recognized under state law can act on the patient's behalf.[11]

The concept of *patient autonomy* was the second lesson to be learned from *Quinlan* and *Cruzan*. Autonomous decision making incorporates the individual's personal values and moral independence without any undue influence. I'm not sure the public noticed that Karen Ann Quinlan lived for another nine years after removal of the ventilator because Mr. Quinlan chose to keep the feeding tube in place. That decision was made in keeping with Karen Ann's religious beliefs, which meant honoring the directive of the Catholic Church concerning the use of artificial nutrition and hydration. Whether you or I would make the same decision is not relevant. Mr. Quinlan's role as guardian obliged him to respect Karen Ann's autonomous values as well as her right to informed consent.

Patient autonomy was also at issue in the 2005 case of Theresa Marie Schiavo. The 41-year-old Florida woman had been in a permanent vegetative state for 15 years when she came to our attention. The legal dispute centered on whether Theresa's medical prognosis triggered the Florida law permitting her husband to remove her feeding tube, in keeping with Theresa's previously stated wishes. Ultimately, Theresa's family was unable to prove that she was not irreversibly unconscious and could be rehabilitated. Theresa Marie Schiavo died on March 31, 2005, 13 days after the withdrawal of artificial nutrition.[12]

The 1976 rallying cry "*It's wrong to keep the patient alive*" and the 2005 chorus of voices chanting "*It's wrong to let the patient die*" are strikingly dissimilar. Yet that wide diversity of opinion illustrates the essential nature of patient autonomy. Health literacy is key to respecting each patient's unique beliefs, preferences and priorities, while ensuring that medical decisions are made by a patient or proxy who has access to reliable and complete information.

The landmark legal cases have focused on medical decision making for incapacitated persons who are terminally ill or irreversibly unconscious. That is in sharp contrast to most patients' reality. Three out of four Americans aged 65 and older and two-thirds of Medicare patients are plagued by multiple chronic medical conditions, which are physical or mental illnesses that last a year or longer, require ongoing medical attention and/or limit the patient's daily living activities. Common examples are COPD, depression, fibromyalgia, diabetes, heart disease, cancer and dementia.[13] That means regular interaction with the health care system and years of making life-altering decisions about treatment, therapy, lifestyle and caregiving. Frequent and recurrent decision making. Nevertheless, the right to informed consent remains constant, no matter what the medical circumstances may be.

One cannot make informed medical decisions without first being informed. Furthermore, the right to informed consent is premised on the distinctive beliefs and values held by each one of us—that's the definition of patient autonomy. Together, they are the legal cornerstones of health literacy. To protect those rights, you must prepare in advance for medical decision making by considering the personal preferences and priorities that are critical to *you*—not to the person in the bed down the hall or your Aunt Fannie when she had the same diagnosis or, quite frankly, your primary care physician.

All you need now are the means to do that.

CHAPTER THREE

The building blocks of health literacy

The fundamental goal of achieving health literacy is to have a process to preserve the right to informed consent and patient autonomy well ahead of any need to use it. That's the only way to ensure that physician, patient, proxy—and attorney—are all speaking the same language when it comes to informed medical decision making. Health literacy has a solid foundation of three building blocks, all rooted in effective communication: resources, shared decision making and action steps.

Building Block A — Health literacy resources

These are the tools you need to access, process and understand reliable health care information and the services needed to make informed decisions in a particular health care situation.

Building Block B - Shared decision making

Shared decision making is a step-by-step communication process for sharing the patient's perspective, gathering needed information and then thoughtfully considering options before granting informed consent.

Building Block C — Action steps

These are specific tasks and documentation to be completed ahead of time in order to fully achieve health literacy and to be prepared for future health care situations—routine or emergency.

- **Chapter Four** addresses the myriad of health care resources now available, including how to tell the good from the not-so-good and how best to learn more about terminology, providers, symptoms, treatments and medications.
- **Chapter Five** is about having and being a health care advocate. That can be anyone from an appointment buddy to a court-appointed guardian, which means this chapter also includes the basics of Advance Care Planning.

- **Chapter Six** concerns choosing the members of your health care provider team, with a focus on the patient-primary care provider relationship.
- **Chapter Seven** covers one of the most important elements of health literacy, the practice of shared decision making. It's an information-gathering and communication tool that applies to everything from choosing health insurance to making funeral arrangements.
- **Chapter Eight** is about one type of advocacy that deserves its own chapter; it's caregiving, whether looking out for someone else or planning ahead for yourself.
- **Chapter Nine** covers proactive care through preventive medicine, with tests and procedures for early detection and healthy living.
- **Chapter Ten** provides a view of the potential harm of overprescribing medications, how to manage multiple prescriptions and how to be a responsible and medication literate patient.
- **Chapter Eleven** is devoted to recognizing when urgent care and emergency care are appropriate and the unique challenges they present for decision making.
- **Chapter Twelve** addresses what is often the most difficult test of shared decision making: facing an unexpected critical health care decision.
- **Chapter Thirteen** is about the extraordinary specialty of palliative care and its potential role in all areas of medicine, from pediatrics to hospice care.
- **Chapter Fourteen** covers the process of dying and the role of advocacy to the very end of life—sometimes even after death—in honoring the patient's right to informed consent and autonomy.
- **Chapter Fifteen** includes the **Good-To-Meet-You-&-In-Case-of-Emergency Profile**, part of the documentation needed for full and effective communication of your emergency information, medical history and care preferences.
- There is also a **Glossary** and an **Appendix** that indexes common decision making dilemmas and how to address them. And I always like to include other sources that I've found to be informational or inspirational, so this book ends with **Recommended Reading** and **Endnotes**.

Now let's get to work.

CHAPTER FOUR

༄༅

Accessing health literacy resources

What a difference a century makes. The *trajectory* of any disease or medical condition is its path or progression from the time of onset to death caused by it. When an illness is likely to be the direct cause of a person's future death, it is a *life-limiting illness*. One hundred years ago, the trajectory of a life-limiting illness was about the same as what we now consider a sudden, unexpected passing: three days.[14] Hardly time to say goodbye. Unlike the early 1900s, today the course of a life-limiting or chronic disease can span years; the diagnosis may be only the beginning of a lengthy journey of decision making. We have demanded more cures and life-extending treatments from researchers and providers and—good news for us—they have delivered in a big way. The flip side is that we're so accustomed to having effective therapies for our urgent, emergency and chronic health conditions that we've stopped being concerned with the details. The problem with that attitude? The devil is in the details.

You can choose to leave all decision making to the professionals or you can commit to being an engaged member of your health care team. The latter is a notion that many people dodge at all costs—but not you, right? To be a fully involved and informed partner in the patient-provider partnership, you must recognize when, how and where to access the tools needed to effectively communicate.

The language of health literacy

Plumbers and engineers and health care providers each have language unique to their vocations. What makes health care exceptional is that—unlike choosing between bronze and chrome shower heads—whether communication is effective may govern whether and how long the customer lives.

Besides the unique nature of medical-speak, there are also common words that have a different meaning in a health care setting. For example, as a writer, negative feedback is bad for me; but in medical tests, negative results are usually a good thing. When it comes to terminology, if you don't have the health literacy equivalent of a secret decoder ring, mistakes are going to be made. You'll find a Glossary of common health care terms in the back of this book. It isn't meant to be an exhaustive medical dictionary, but it does cover language you are likely to come across in the process of medical decision making. It's worth a quick read-through, if only as a refresher or to clarify any misconceptions you may have.

This guy walks into an emergency room . . .

To illustrate how crucial the meaning of words can be, let me tell you about a series of studies being conducted with emergency room doctors. They are presented with a hypothetical patient who has a Living Will stating he wants no life prolonging measures if a triggering event of either terminal illness or permanent unconsciousness occurs.

Then the doctors are asked how they would "code" the man (what medical care they would provide) when he starts having chest pains and difficulty breathing. Only 22 percent say the patient should have "full code" status, meaning he receives all possible life-saving and resuscitation care. The remaining doctors answer that they would *not* treat the symptoms of his heart attack, but would provide comfort care only. That's because they mistakenly think a Living Will is the same as a Do Not Resuscitate medical order (DNR) and they mistakenly think a DNR order means to provide comfort care only.[15]

These providers have an alarming lack of health literacy on several levels: 1) the terms of the Living Will do not apply until a triggering event occurs; 2) a Living Will is *not* a medical order; 3) a DNR is a medical order to forego resuscitation efforts only if a person's heart and breathing have both stopped; and 4) every patient should receive emergency medical care until he is either stable or has died. These study results are a chilling example of medical term confusion. Accessing reliable health care information and being familiar with the language of health care are both vital to health literacy. Whether it's the patient or the provider, somebody in the room has to get it right.

What is a "health care provider"?

You may notice I use the term "provider," rather than "physician" or "doctor." That's because the tenets of health literacy apply anytime and anywhere you are receiving health care, regardless of the title or degree of the person delivering those services. So, to name just a few, "provider" includes a registered nurse; physician's assistant; occupational, speech or physical therapist; nurse practitioner; surgical technician; licensed or practical nurse; pharmacist or pharmacy technician; nurse's aid or certified nursing assistant; emergency medical technician (EMT); home health care aide; radiology or phlebotomy (blood) technician; and a physician of any specialty, such as family practice, geriatrics or psychiatry. Anytime you are immersed in the health care system, your rights to informed consent and autonomy remain intact.

Consider making the Internet a member of your team

Nothing matches the scope and convenience of the Internet. Your local library has neither the space nor the funds to keep in circulation all the relevant health care information now available. However, they may have public terminals in case you don't have personal access to a computer, tablet or smartphone. Find someone to give you basic research guidance, join an adult education class on Internet surfing or make friends with the nearest teenager. With more than half of American adults having used the World Wide Web to look up health topics,[16] we can safely say the Internet is not a passing fancy.

Right up front, I'll share the same caveat found in every website's fine print: *Information you get on the Internet is not a substitute for being seen in person by a health care professional.* However, as well as being an amazing repository of information, the Web is also a portal to traditional resources: agency phone numbers, local providers, relevant books or even where to find real live human beings with needed expertise. For example: online I found a SHIIP (Senior Health Insurance Information Program) community seminar where I could ask questions about Medicare and talk to others about what they had learned; I narrowed down my choices for a primary care physician on the Web and then showed the list to other providers and friends for recommendations; after viewing official drug information for a new prescription online, I spoke to my pharmacist about any anecdotal feedback she has gotten from customers.

These are just some of the topics you can become familiar with or learn about in detail on health care websites:

- Medical terms
- Medication and supplements
- Preventive tests and procedures
- Diseases and conditions
- Home health care resources
- Medical treatments, clinical trials and medical devices
- Location and credentials of providers
- Advance Care Planning

Approach Internet sources as you would any other provider of products or services: with cautious optimism and a commitment to ask the right questions up front.

Searching on the Internet for health care information

Think of an Internet search engine as an index for the world's most ginormous encyclopedia. You enter one or more keyword searches and it reveals every website, photo, vendor, video and news article that has ever mentioned that word or phrase— or any variation of it—in the history of the Internet. I happen to favor Google (www.Google.com.), but there are many search engines available; over time most folks settle on the one they like the best. In entering your keyword search, try to think like a computer programmer, who is spending his life trying to think like you: *What words or phrases ("keywords") first come to mind relating to this issue?* The more specific you are, the more likely you will zero in on what you're looking for.

If you want to know what preventive care tests you should have and how often, search *"chart of recommended regular preventive medical tests"* or *"preventive medical tests AND older Americans."* Most search engines have options to narrow results by category type and date. For instance, to find charts, you can ask for "images" over the past 12 months, although that is *not* a guarantee that all results are less than a year old, so pay attention to the date on sources. Also, the ranking of search results is not a measure of accuracy or even popularity.

Examples of keyword search phrases:
"looking for a [specialist] in [city]"
"health care issues when travelling to [country]"
"most successful [smoking cessation/weight loss] programs"
"side effects of [drug name] AND available research"
As you gaze upon the 1,297,420 results that just appeared, now what?

Who can you really trust these days?

The information superhighway is an invaluable source of health care knowledge that complements—but does not replace—the expertise of the provider team I have mindfully assembled. Plumbers, engineers and providers are not all equal, and neither are websites. Here are my common sense rules for using the Web:

Rule #1: *Appearing on the Internet does not make something true.* That also goes for information printed on high gloss card stock.

Rule #2: *Some sources are more reliable than others.* Being for-profit is not a deal breaker, but if you cannot find the health care information for all the advertisements popping up or blocking your field of vision, move on.

Rule #3: *Outdated health care information is a deal breaker.* Every article should have a date of original publication. Years are like light years in many fields of medical research, so look for the most recent source.

Rule #4: *Verifiable implies reliable.* Does the site identify the source of all information (experts or organizations)? If there are no References or Endnotes to validate facts, figures or research results, then run, don't walk to the next site. If you want to go full-geek, click through and read the original source.

Rule #5: *More is better.* Even if you find a website you like, don't hesitate to shop around, especially if you are seeking information on treatment options. Compare dates of publication, the citations relied on and the level of detail to judge the most useful source.

Rule #6: *A chat room is a chat room, even if it's part of a legitimate health care website.* Many sites include a "message board," which is nothing more than a cyber soapbox. It may or may not be subject to editorial scrutiny and it is virtually impossible to distinguish between frustrated patients, legitimate providers and angry people in jammies.

The online resources mentioned throughout this book are included because I consider them dependable and user-friendly, but for *any* resource you consult in print or online, do your own due diligence on its reliability. Visit *Trust It or Trash It* (http://www.trustortrash.org) or the *National Institutes of Health* site (https://ods.od.nih.gov - Evaluating Health Information) for tips on evaluating trustworthiness. Websites morph and even change ownership over time, so these are not permanent recommendations, nor do I have any affiliation with any of them (except for my own websites, which are listed in the back of the book).

The health care websites I recommend

[If you are reading a digital version of this book, all references are hyperlinked so you can click through to the source. For the print version, simply go to the website shown and then enter the specific subject matter in the site's internal search function. For example, for www.hopkinsmedicine.org - Screening Tests for Common Diseases, you would go to the www.hopkinsmedicine.org website and search for "*screening tests for common diseases.*"]

- https://medlineplus.gov (Medline Plus) - This site is sponsored by the National Institutes of Health and the U.S. National Library of Medicine, both part of the U.S. Department of Health & Human Services (HHS). Good for finding **providers** and for

healthy living tips, it has a directory of old-school contacts for health care resources.

- www.cdc.gov (Centers for Disease Control and Prevention) - Also part of HHS, the focus is on **statistics and data**. It also has health information for **travelers**, **public health warnings** and the ever-popular feature, "Disease of the Week."
- www.mayoclinic.org (Mayo Clinic) - I consider this the most consumer-friendly of health care sites. It covers the gambit of topics from **medical terms** to **medical devices** and everything in between.
- www.webmd.com (WebMD) - Part of the WebMD Network, this is a comprehensive health care site for the public. Two sister sites are www.medicinenet.com, which has a solid **glossary** plus more in-depth articles; and www.medscape.com, whose target audience is health care professionals. (Don't let that stop you—register to access all of MedScape's features.)
- https://clinicaltrials.gov - A function of the U.S. National Institutes of Health (HHS), it is dedicated to information about **clinical trials** and experimental drug therapy trial studies.
- http://healthfinder.gov (HHS) - Good source for **healthy living** guides and general information on specific **diseases and conditions**.

Specialty resources

If you want in-depth detail about a specific disease or medical condition, I encourage you to also visit one or more of the websites focused on that disorder. Many are sponsored by organizations started by folks like you who wanted to know more about the medical condition afflicting them or a loved one. Just three examples:
- **Alzheimer's Disease:** www.alz.org - The Alzheimer's Association[17] or www.alzheimer.ca/en - The Alzheimer's Association of Canada.
- **Cancer:** www.cancer.org - The American Cancer Society or www.cancer.net - The American Society of Clinical Oncology.
- **Heart disease and strokes:** www.strokeassociation.org - The American Stroke Association and www.heart.org – The American Heart Association (the two are now joined into one organization).
- For a **pill identifier** feature (by color, shape and markings), go to https://pillbox.nlm.nih.gov (The National Library of Medicine) or http://reference.medscape.com (Medscape).

Consider whether there may be specialized care or resources available due to a patient's unique characteristics, such as age, level of income or former military service. For example, geriatricians specialize in diseases and care issues unique to aging and elderly patients; the Veterans' Health Administration has programs to address health issues caused by, or exacerbated by, military service. Doesn't it make sense to see the provider who knows the most about you and your health care issue?

For *any* medical condition or treatment option, go to your favorite search engine and enter the search terms, *"best websites for [medical condition],"* then work your way down the list. When you later speak with your provider face-to-face—which you should do—ask for other recommendations. You might get the big eye roll or you might get a great lead.

You know who else you can trust?

In preparing to write this chapter, I thought back on where I've gotten some of the best health care information, referrals and functional wisdom. Duh, my friends. My inner circle—I call them *The Two Percent Club*—are some of the savviest people I know when it comes to medical issues. Only one has a health care-related background, but all of them are self-educated on the information they need because that's what the circumstances demand. Period. They are perceptive and curious and exceptionally responsible about being fully informed about their own care and that of the people they watch over. They continue to be an invaluable resource in maintaining my own health literacy.

Along with seeking your providers' expertise, don't hesitate to ask family members and friends what they learned in any health care situation similar to yours and what they might do differently, if they could. Albert Einstein, a pretty brainy guy himself, said it best: *"The only source of knowledge is experience."*

Health Literacy Rules of the Road

Health literacy is dependent on gathering reliable information and then using it to make informed and autonomous medical decisions. Here are my simple rules to keep patient and provider focused on those essential elements of health literacy.

Patients' Health Literacy Rules of the Road

- You have the right to be fully informed before granting autonomous consent for a medical procedure. Anyone who says different is wrong.
- If you already know what you're going to discuss with your provider, take a list of questions with you—written down, not in your head.
- Take along an "appointment buddy" to any important medical consultation to act as another set of ears, an additional source of questions and a notetaker.
- Ask for clarification. If you're uncomfortable saying, *"I have no idea what that means,"* get over it. Learn all you can about all medical treatment alternatives, from taking a new prescription to accepting that it's time for hospice care.
- Anything important enough to be in writing is important enough to be understood before you sign it. *"Don't worry, nobody knows what this means"* is not an explanation.
- Do not let a patient-provider conversation end until you verify whether there is another step to be taken, who is going to take it and when.
- If you're not entirely sure you have all the information you need or fully understand what you've heard, ask who to call after you leave. When you wake up in the middle of the night with a question, write it down.
- A health literate patient-provider relationship is based on trust, and trust is a two-way street. Be honest when sharing your symptoms and health concerns. Providers have amazing talents but being clairvoyant is not typically one of them (if only).
- Give providers permission to be honest, even if the news is bad, the condition can no longer be treated or it's time to talk about end-of-life care.
- Promise yourself that your answer to the question *"Well, what did you find out?"* will never again be *"I don't know, the doctor didn't say."*

- The only way to identify a patient's autonomous priorities and preferences is to learn about the patient's unique journey.
- For effective patient communication, you don't need to use small words, simply take a moment to explain what the big words mean.
- A video or a flip chart with cartoon characters may or may not enhance communication, but making eye contact with the patient instead of with your computer screen definitely will.
- If a patient asks a question, he is probably willing to hear your complete and honest answer, which he needs to make a fully informed decision.
- Even if they don't tell you often enough—or at all—your patients are grateful for all you do. Yes, they want to believe that you can perform miracles, but in their hearts, they know you are doing the best a human being can do.
- When you can no longer offer your patient a cure, please trust that they understand it is not because you do not care or because you have given up on them. If you doubt whether they know that, tell them.
- Even if you can no longer treat the disease, continue to treat the patient by practicing shared decision making concerning all available care options.
- If you can accept that life will one day come to an end for every one of your patients, it will help them to do the same.

CHAPTER FIVE

The crucial role of health care advocacy

Champion, supporter, backer, proponent, spokesperson, fighter, crusader, booster. Those labels are all synonymous with being an *advocate*, one who speaks for or intercedes on behalf of another person. Considering the challenges of managing one's health care, I would welcome any one of those archetypes on my team, wouldn't you?

Along with advancements in treatment, the past few decades have brought big changes in how health care is delivered. I had a kidney stone in the 1980s and was hospitalized for three days, just waiting for that little rascal to either dissolve or appear. Fast forward 30 years and I know someone who underwent a mastectomy in outpatient surgery. Nowadays, you are not hospitalized unless you are really sick, and with staff shortages, you need someone to be your voice, assess your discomfort and get assistance when needed. Then there's the biggie: requiring someone to speak for you because you've lost all decision making capacity. That's the continuum of advocacy: from an appointment buddy to a court-ordered guardian.

Before we go any further, never discount the value of the advocate in waiting, the person who knows you best and is there for you, no matter what. Yes, I'm talking about *you*, my friend. Being your own health care advocate as long as you have the capacity is Job One and achieving health literacy will make that possible. Still, it's prudent to plan for situations when you need either just a bit of support or someone to act as your full-time substitute decision maker.

An appointment buddy

Were you ever in a doctor's office and wished you had someone with you? You know, to ask the question you didn't think of until three a.m. the following morning? Then there was the time you just didn't feel like being alone afterwards.

I call that someone an *appointment buddy*. It can be a friend, a family member or even a kindhearted neighbor. Whether or not you're comfortable having that person present during a patient-provider consultation, occasionally you just need friendly transportation and someone to listen on the way home. Consider a reciprocal arrangement to do the same for another person and start thinking now who might be willing and able to fill that role if needed in the future.

A reminder here that cell phones can also be a means to three-way communication: Put that long-distance family member on the speaker while you consult with your provider. They will hear the conversation first-hand and can chime in with questions of their own. Of course, respectfully first seek the provider's consent.

Hospital sitter or patient companion

A *hospital sitter* or *patient companion* is a specialized aide who stays with a hospitalized patient with dementia or any condition that requires full-time monitoring. Some hospitals provide this service upon request or a sitter can be hired at the patient's cost. (There may be Medicaid assistance in some states.) Companions are present to ensure the patient's physical safety and to alert staff of needed care or of an emergency. They do not typically provide hands-on caregiving.

Professional patient advocate

Even if you have a family member or friend willing to accompany you to appointments, explore treatment options with you and speak up when you're speechless, if they are too far away or just don't feel qualified, what's an alternative? You can hire a *professional patient advocate* to make sure health care providers are acting in your best interests. They are also there to convey information to you, the patient, or to your decision maker, as each situation warrants. Professional patient advocates are paid to be an extra pair of ears, to ask the right questions and to make sure the patient's wishes are honored.

Depending on patient needs, duties may include filing insurance claims, tracking appointments, researching treatments, arranging for home care and purchasing medical equipment. The patient advocate's fees, usually charged by the hour, are not covered by health insurance or Medicare and will be the responsibility of the patient.

An appointed health care proxy

Capacity is the mental ability to understand the nature and consequences of an issue, make a decision regarding it and comprehend the effects of that choice. Presently you still have full decision making capacity and can manage your health care, but that could change. This is the time to answer a very important question: *"If I am ever too ill to think or speak for myself, who do I want to speak for me?"* You have the opportunity now to name someone as your substitute decision maker, a *health care proxy*, and appoint that person in a written Durable Power of Attorney for Health Care, which is one type of Health Care Advance Directive.

If hospitalized, you are likely to be treated by providers who have never met you before: emergency care personnel, a specialist, an intensivist and/or a hospitalist (who attends to other doctors' hospitalized patients). As you will learn in Chapter Seven, one of the most important elements of shared decision making is the provider's understanding of the patient's values, preferences and priorities. If the patient is unable to communicate, it's the proxy's duty to supply that context. The best choice as proxy is a person who knows what the patient would choose, will honor the patient's autonomous choices, will stand up to medical professionals, will ask the tough questions and will make the hard calls, if necessary.

The adage that *"80 percent of success is showing up"* definitely applies to a health care proxy, so it should be someone who can be present in an emergency. Name a backup, in case the first proxy is unable to serve, but avoid appointing two or more as co-proxies—ruling by committee can leave the patient dangling in decision limbo.

In addition to being an all-around advocate for the patient, a health care proxy should be prepared to perform any or all of the following duties:

- Meet with health care providers to get information and to make a treatment plan.
- Seek specialists and get second opinions.
- Consent to, refuse to consent to or withdraw consent for all medical treatments.
- Arrange for hospitalization, rehabilitation, home care or hospice care.
- Review medical records and consent to their appropriate disclosure to others.
- Take steps to ensure that all insurance and assistance benefits are received.

The duties of a health care proxy do *not* include hands-on caregiving and financial responsibility for the patient. If you want someone to manage assets, you need a separate Durable Power of Attorney for Financial Matters. There are lots of details to consider, so I recommend visiting a competent elder law or estate planning attorney to get it all right.

For a variety of reasons, the emergency room is *not* the place for your proxy to learn of his appointment. First, every person deserves to consider whether to serve and, secondly, a proxy cannot effectively advocate for unknown care preferences. With that in mind, once you've narrowed your choices:

- Have a crucial conversation in which you fully explain the proxy's duties and responsibilities. Share your own answer to the question, *"When do you think enough is enough?"* and talk in detail about the use of life prolonging measures and a decision making process for unexpected circumstances.
- Ask your potential proxy the question *"If I am unable to make medical decisions*

in the future, are you willing to act as my proxy and honor my wishes for care?"

• Once your nominee understands his role as proxy and agrees to serve, document the appointment in a Health Care Advance Directive that complies with state law.

The proxy's decision making authority begins when you lose decision making capacity. If you regain the ability to self-manage your care—whether that is waking up after surgery or being successfully rehabilitated after a stroke—your proxy is no longer in charge.

A proxy-by-statute or surrogate decision maker

In reality, when a decision needs to be made about the care of an incapacitated patient, health care providers usually turn to the family member who happens to be present. That's to be expected. It's efficient, it's nonconfrontational and it's appropriate most of the time. When that system doesn't work is when there is a disagreement over the patient's treatment plan or there is no one willing or able to act as the patient's substitute decision maker. State laws address that potential challenge.

If the patient has executed an advance directive (a Living Will) covering the use of life prolonging measures, those instructions should always guide providers. If there is no Living Will and no appointed health care proxy, state laws specify a pecking order of those eligible to be recognized as a *proxy-by-statute* or *surrogate decision maker*. The list usually starts with a guardian, then the spouse, adult children, adult siblings and so on down the line. The glitch in these statutory solutions is that they don't kick in until the patient is either terminal or irreversibly unconscious, so a proxy-by-statute is not recognized to make the many care decisions that can arise long before the end of life is approaching. Also, with few exceptions, states do not recognize anyone not related to the patient, such as a long-time domestic partner, BFF or beloved sister-in-law. Grandchildren qualify as surrogates in less than a third.

If you fail to appoint a health care proxy ahead of time, you may end up with a surrogate decision maker you would rather not have. Worse yet, if you have no family available to step in, decision making may come to a screeching halt or be contrary to your preferences. Preserving the right to consent with an appointed proxy is a use-it-or-lose-it proposition. If you have not already, start thinking about your options now, as you work your way toward Chapter Fifteen.

A guardianship

A guardianship is a court-ordered relationship in which the guardian acts on behalf of a person lacking decision making competency, the ward. The legal process of establishing a guardianship takes time and money, so it is not a practical solution for medical decision making on a temporary basis or in an emergency. And just to add to the drama, in about half of the states, when a patient has both an appointed health care proxy and a subsequent court-appointed guardian, the proxy can overrule the guardian in conflicts over the use of life prolonging measures.

Many states have "standby guardianships" by which a person who is still competent names a contingent guardian, specifying the mental or physical conditions that trigger the appointment. If the time ever comes, filing the petition is a simple procedure and this process guarantees the appointment of a guardian who was hand-picked by the ward.

Volunteer or professional guardians

To address the needs of the estimated 20 percent of Americans aged 65 and older who are "elder orphans,"[18] every state now has some form of public program to protect those without anyone to oversee their care. The guardian may be an agency or an unpaid volunteer individual. Another alternative is a professional guardian, an industry that has flourished to fill the need unmet by public guardian agencies and volunteers. Individuals and non-profit and for-profit agencies act as guardian for a fee, paid from the ward's assets. The level of certification, background checks and oversight for either alternative is a function of each state's statutory regulation, if any.

Guidance for proxy decision making

Whether it's a patient-appointed proxy, a proxy-by-statute or a court-appointed guardian, a substitute decision maker should be guided by the following principles before granting informed consent, in this order of priority:

• Refer to the patient's previous clear-cut verbal statements or written instructions in a Health Care Advance Directive, if available.

• Use substituted judgment by inferring what the patient would do under the circumstances if he were able, relying on specific or general evidence of the patient's values, attitudes about life in general and views on how life is meant to be lived.

• Do what is in the best interest of the patient when there is no trustworthy evidence of what the patient would want.

• Withhold a treatment if it would be inhumane to continue the treatment.

• In the case of whether to remove a life prolonging measure, err on the side of preserving life if no other position can be supported.[19]

Decision making (by others) after you pass away

By definition, the proxy's authority to make health care decisions ends once the patient dies. Realistically, decision making may extend beyond the patient's passing concerning two issues: organ donation and disposition of remains (including authorization for an autopsy).

If you wish to be an organ donor, first complete your state's donor registry and then clearly communicate your wishes to loved ones, verbally and in writing. Under federal law, if a patient registers as an organ donor and/or specifies his wish to be a donor in written directives, that consent cannot be withheld by survivors.[20] If you *don't* want to be an organ donor, that should be clearly stated, verbally and in writing.

As for decisions about having an autopsy, disposition of the body and memorial or funeral rituals, some state laws dictate who has legal authority to make those decisions and whether the deceased's wishes must be in writing, so check with a local attorney. As with many matters relating to the end of life, your survivors will be forever grateful for any preplanning you do. The reassurance of knowing one is carrying out the deceased's wishes will be as appreciated as being relieved of the decision making burden.

CHAPTER SIX

୫୦ଓଃ

Assembling a health care team

Conspicuous by their absence from the previous chapter on advocacy are those who will have the most influence—other than you—on whether your health care experiences are positive or negative, productive or frustrating, restorative or detrimental: your health care providers. Assembling a team of individuals with the skills, availability and compassion you deserve who will be there for you in any health care situation is not a duty to be taken lightly.

A primary care provider is the health care professional you visit most often, whether that is a general practitioner, family practitioner, internist, physician's assistant or nurse practitioner. Your primary care provider performs your annual checkup, is often the first person to detect and diagnose a health care issue and the person most likely to refer you to a specialist, such as a podiatrist, gynecologist or cardiologist. For children, it may be a pediatrician, just as a geriatrician may fill that role for an aging person. If you have a chronic medical condition, the specialist for that disorder may take on the role of your primary care provider, practically speaking. Each patient's situation is unique.

In reviewing these questions, consider that many of them also apply to other affiliated providers, such as a pharmacist, dentist, massage therapist, social worker, home health care aide, physical or occupational therapist or even a hospital. And never forget that the receptionist, office manager and nurse are often the portal to the provider—they are important members of your team as well.

The practical considerations

Over a health care lifetime, you will face one or more of these circumstances:
- Choosing a provider for the first time as an emancipated adult.
- Moving to a new community.
- Adjusting to the retirement of your long-time primary care provider.
- Seeking a specialist for a new medical issue.
- Knowing in your heart that it's time for a change.

If your search for a health care professional begins with the Yellow Pages or Google, your eyes will soon be glazing over. Let's apply some narrowing criteria first:
- Visit www.Medicare.gov - Find & compare doctors, hospitals & other providers to search by zip code. For other health insurers, ask for a list of the accepted network providers in your area.
- Consider the type of patient-provider relationship you prefer, and be honest with yourself: shared decision making or the paternalistic somebody-please-tell-me-what-to-do style? Friendly, conversational manner or formal interaction?
- Will you be seeing this doctor for one or more existing medical conditions or to establish a patient-provider relationship for future needs?
- Can you seek a recommendation from another provider? Don't be afraid to ask: *"Who's your doctor, doc?"* or *"Would you send your loved one to this provider?"*
- Ask your friends who they see, whether they would recommend them and *why* (what they look for in a provider may be very different from your priorities).
- If you know a practicing nurse, ask for input.
- Is the provider accepting new patients right now?
- Where is the provider's office located and can you get there easily with available transportation? Is there ample and accessible parking?
- Will the provider accept your health insurance coverage and process the claims?
- How many years of experience does the provider have? Visit www.certificationmatters.org to verify the board certifications held by a provider.
- What is the provider's experience in treating any existing conditions you have?
- Is the provider in a large practice? If your provider is ever unavailable, can you be seen by an associate and are you willing to do that?
- How old is the provider? At the risk of being an ageist, I strive to have providers who will be around at least as long as I will. As a matter of fact, one of my specialists just announced her retirement. A bit early, if you ask me, which no one did.

Who is that masked stranger in the white coat?

A friend and I were recently searching on the Web to locate a specialist we thought had joined our community. In that process, we were shocked to discover all the people implying that they are medical practitioners by using the title of "Doctor" when, in fact, they hold an academic degree in a not-found-in-Webster's specialty. Believe me, I'm all about alternative treatment methods, I'm just not hip to insinuating that someone is a doctor of medicine unless that person has actually attended medical school. And graduated. Here's the lesson: Verify the credentials of any health care provider—or alleged health care provider—you are considering. Read the fine print,

...ter to a medical dictionary and then check with your state board of medicine to confirm licensing.

Plan now for what tomorrow may bring

When choosing a provider, consider possible future issues and ask about the provider's policy on the following:
- What hospitals is the provider affiliated with? Are the hospitals conveniently located and are you comfortable with those options?
- Does the provider use a hospitalist for his hospitalized patients? If so, who is it? How is provider-hospitalist communication coordinated?
- Are evening or weekend appointments possible? Can the provider or his associates be reached when the office is closed?
- Is the provider affiliated with an urgent care clinic for treatment outside regular office hours? If not, where should you go for urgent (non-emergency) care?
- What type of medical conditions would the provider refer to a specialist and what would he treat himself?
- Is the provider in a multi-discipline clinic that includes other specialists and services?
- How will the provider handle communication with an outside specialist?
- Will your primary care provider have access to your medical tests and records at other practitioners as part of a provider network? (Remind me to tell you the story of the physical therapist who saved the day for me.)
- What diagnostics, e.g., radiology, blood tests, colonoscopy or mammography, is the provider able to conduct and evaluate in-house?

Meeting face-to-face

You can request an "interview" appointment with a prospective provider. Ask your health insurer what, if any, cost there will be to you for that time. Whether you go that route or wait until you need to see the provider for the first time (there's always the yearly physical or the Medicare Annual Wellness Visit to get things rolling), you should observe or ask questions to learn the following:
- Are the office facilities clean and located in a safe setting?
- Is the office staff friendly, courteous and respectful of you and other patients?
- How long can you expect to wait to get an appointment once you call?
- For urgent medical care, can you see someone within a day?
- If you call with a question, how quickly can you expect to get a call back?

- Does the provider use online communication (appointment scheduling, reminders, test results, etc.)? If you want old-school methods, are they available?
- If there is a language barrier, does the practice have access to a translator?
- Once you meet the provider, do you feel valued as a patient? Are you allowed to tell about yourself and to get any immediate questions fully answered?
- Does anything about that first visit make you uncomfortable? Listen to the little voice in the back of your head. This is a very important decision.

What to bring to your first meeting

There is a role for you to play in forging this new relationship. Under HIPAA, you have a right to a copy of your medical records, so once you've made a firm decision, make sure your new provider can access your previous medical records. If not, authorize all former or existing providers and specialists to transmit a copy of your medical records to the new provider. Be prepared to complete a new patient questionnaire, which means you will need what I like to call your **Good-To-Meet-You-&-In-Case-of-Emergency Profile** (more detail about this in Chapter Fifteen). Be prepared to recount the dates of prior major surgeries and illnesses.

You're starting a new relationship with someone who may play a critical role in your life going forward. If you do your homework, you'll be just fine. Take a deep breath, smile and welcome the value of a fresh perspective on your health care.

CHAPTER SEVEN

ଔଓ

The art of shared decision making

You just got an unexpected diagnosis or a call that a loved one is in the emergency room with a possible stroke or your doctor is considering a major lifestyle change—for *you*. You need to evaluate options and make very important decisions, maybe even on the fly—choices that could have deep and lasting effects on you or someone you love. You know what you need? A clear-cut process for communicating and decision making in which the health care provider fully appreciates the patient's perspective and the patient or decision maker fully understands his available treatment options before making a choice.

Lucky for us, what we need already exists. In fact, it's been around since 1982, when the term was first coined in a Presidential commission on bioethics working toward improving physician-patient communication and informed consent in health care.[21] It's called *shared decision making*. Although its greatest value is in critical medical situations—such as designing a treatment plan for a life-limiting diagnosis, committing to long-term rehabilitation or considering a major lifestyle change—it can be an invaluable tool whenever you face health care-related alternatives.

It seems we're at cross purposes when it comes to patient-provider communication: Providers don't think their patients want to participate in decision making and patients want more information than they usually get.[22] This is not good. Properly implemented, shared decision making achieves the goal of bringing these parallel ways of thinking into alignment. That's because by its very nature, it encourages both patient and provider to be consciously involved in the steps that lead to informed decision making.

Practicing shared decision making

We're about to go into a lot more detail, but this will get us started. Keep in mind that this process applies whether care is being managed by the patient or by a substitute decision maker. Following here are the basics elements of shared decision making.

Shared decision making

I. The provider clearly communicates a summary of the diagnosis, medical condition or health care concern that requires decision making.

II. The provider learns as much as possible about the patient, including the patient's personal and treatment goals.

III. The provider offers the treatment or care options available to achieve the patient's goals, keeping in mind the patient's values, preferences and priorities.

IV. The provider and the patient (or substitute decision maker) fully discuss and consider available options for care or treatment.

V. The patient or decision maker grants informed consent to proceed with a procedure or treatment plan.[23]

Now let's view shared decision making step-by-step, expanding on the purpose of each crucial component. Whether you are the patient, substitute decision maker or provider, pay attention to the role of *every* player in order to set your expectations for others. Before even the first step is taken, the decision maker—whether that is the patient or a proxy—should embrace his crucial role in decision making, keeping in mind this goal: *shared decision making is the process by which the right to informed consent is preserved.*

I. The provider clearly communicates the health care issue

- Determine if the patient has decision making capacity, and, if not, identify the decision maker and arrange for the decision maker to be present.
- Designate a reliable notetaker in the room, offer a summary of the provider's notes or suggest another means to record key messages.
- Assess whether there is any mental impairment, physical condition or cultural and linguistic barrier that could hamper communication and address it.
- Clearly summarize the diagnosis, medical condition or health care concern that requires decision making.
- Define medical terminology as needed, explain common terms that may be confusing to the lay person and spell easily misunderstood terms.
- Use models or diagrams, as the health care issue requires.
- Explain whether additional tests are needed to make a firm diagnosis and, if so, how, when and where they will be done and when results will be available.
- Explain the likely course of events, or various courses if more than one outcome is possible; provide probabilities, as appropriate, in easy-to-understand formats;

include the likely outcome if no action is taken.

- Invite the patient or decision maker to ask questions about the diagnosis or issue.
- Use the "teach-back method" to gauge the patient or decision maker's understanding by asking him to repeat what the provider has said, in the patient's or decision maker's own words.

II. The provider learns about the patient

- Review the patient's medical records and have the patient relate his medical history to learn about any relevant existing conditions and guage the patient's previous experience with medical decision making.
- Learn as much as possible about the patient, including the patient's occupation, lifestyle, family situation, dependents, existing network of support and resources, level of mobility, capacity for self-care, social interaction and family history that may impact current health care issues and options for treatment.
- Determine if the patient is currently undergoing medical treatment and how it may be affected by the health care issue at hand.
- Ask what matters most to the patient, including his personal priorities, beliefs and values, cultural influences, spiritual/religious views, personal and treatment goals and the timing of upcoming life events.
- Verify whether the patient has the mental and physical capacity to be a full participant in implementing a treatment plan going forward; if not, identify additional concerned persons and/or decision makers to be included in a discussion about making a treatment plan.
- The provider demonstrates a full understanding of the patient's situation and perspective by repeating back his understanding of what he knows about the patient, in the provider's own words.

III. The provider offers available options

- Review available, reliable and relevant research on treatment options.
- Explain the treatment or care most likely to achieve the patient's personal and treatment goals, keeping in mind the patient's values, preferences and priorities.
- Offer an unbiased view of each treatment option, detailing the benefits and risks of each alternative, possible complications, potential side effects and probabilities.
- Address the consequences of doing nothing or practicing "watchful waiting."
- Clearly define each potential therapy as a pharmaceutical, surgical, invasive or non-invasive procedure.

- Clarify whether each option is meant to cure the underlying disease; to treat symptoms without an intent to cure; to provide palliative or comfort care; or to prolong the patient's life.
- Explain the possible outcomes if there is no cure available, the cure doesn't work or there is a decision to stop the curative treatment.
- Define medical terminology as needed, explaining common terms that may be confusing to the layperson and spelling easily-misunderstood terms for the patient or decision maker.
- From the patient's perspective, address debilitating or toxic side effects; the impact on mobility, capacity and the patient's daily life; in-home or facility caregiving needs; and any costs of services or equipment not covered by insurance.
- Offer other supplemental sources of information on treatment options that may aid the patient (e.g., videos, pamphlets, websites, specialists, support groups).
- Include the input of other providers who may be involved (e.g., specialists, a social worker, a therapist) and explain how communication will be handled.
- Clarify whether and when a treatment decision needs to be made.
- Invite the patient or decision maker to ask questions about the treatment or care options being offered.
- Use the "teach-back method" to gauge the patient or decision maker's understanding by asking him to repeat what the provider has said, in the patient's or decision maker's own words.

IV. The provider and decision maker fully discuss options

- Once available alternatives have been explained, assess whether there may be other parties who need to be consulted before a decision can be made.
- Address any evidence of the decision maker's confusion or distress as a reaction to the diagnosis, the result of a temporary or permanent mental or physical condition or the aftereffects of a procedure or medication.
- Encourage the decision maker to fully explore the possible outcomes of each alternative being considered.
- Acknowledge that the patient or decision maker may need time to consider options and return for further discussion at a follow-up appointment.

V. The patient or decision maker grants informed consent

- The patient or decision maker consents to a specific procedure or treatment and clearly indicates his understanding of the steps to be implemented.

- The provider agrees with the choice, unless there is a question of medical futility or moral opposition to the treatment plan.
- If the provider objects to the decision maker's choice, he encourages further discussion or, as appropriate, refers the patient to another provider.
- The patient or decision maker acknowledges the right to change his mind later and the possible consequences of doing so.
- The provider and decision maker agree on action steps to be taken and a timeline for the treatment plan.
- The provider and decision maker agree on a procedure for re-assessing the situation, ongoing decision making and future follow-up to verify that there is proper implementation and adherence to the plan.

At the risk of stating the obvious . . .

That was slightly mind-melting. In full detail, this process seems daunting, but each health care situation dictates how thorough you need to be. Obviously, having stitches for a minor kitchen mishap doesn't demand the same complex decision making as crafting a treatment plan to battle a diagnosis of cancer.

I never said being health literate would be effortless, or simple. The process of shared decision making exemplifies the core elements of health literacy: information gathering and informed decision making. From preventive care to end-of-life care, informed medical decision making means investing the time and effort to thoughtfully consider available options and then making choices that respect the patient's unique circumstances. It is a process that embraces the patient's story, which is the perspective that only the patient or his trusted advocate can communicate. Then effective shared decision making proceeds to respect the qualities, life experiences and values that makes each patient different from every other patient.

CHAPTER EIGHT

ℬℭ

Caregiving

Caregiving includes any service that assists a person in managing daily life, from having someone run errands to around-the-clock long-term care—and everything in between. Caregiving literacy embraces the same shared decision making process as other health care issues: Openly and honestly evaluate the situation, access and consider available resources based on the person's unique needs and priorities and make an informed decision.

Twenty-nine percent of American adults are taking care of someone who is ill, disabled or aging. Most of these caregivers are uncompensated family members and friends,[24] and caregiving is yet another demographically challenged area of health care. As compared to 60 years ago, we have smaller families and the percentage of one-person households is three times what it was in the 1950s. Those two statistics suggest that those dealing with a chronic disabling illness or the issues of aging today are less likely to have live-in assistance or family members to help. We know this for a fact: Between now and 2030, the number of potential caregivers will grow *one percent* as the number of Americans who need caregiving will increase *79 percent*.[25] That cannot be good.

Evaluating the need for caregiving

If you're concerned about the safety or care needs of a family member or friend, there are self-guiding checklists for evaluating whether it may be time to seek help. Here are two resources:

http://www.caregiverslibrary.org - Needs Assessment
http://www.aarp.org - Assessment Checklist

Admittedly, it is beyond the expertise of most folks to make a comprehensive needs assessment, especially for a close loved one. It can be difficult to ask questions about personal care issues; for someone with a degenerative disease, it's tricky to suggest that independent living is compromised. And even if you are certain there's a need for assistance, can you fully identify all the caregiving options available? It's time to call in an expert who can act with an outsider's objectivity—as well as being the messenger of what may be unwelcome news.

Ask the primary care physician to recommend an agency or individual to make a full care assessment. That includes visiting the home to evaluate safety issues and confirm if modifications can be made. A staff social worker (another health care occupation suffering severe shortages) should evaluate and make caregiving recommendations for any patient being discharged from the hospital. Fully inform the evaluator of the person's background, resources, and personal priorities. Keep these issues in mined when considering options for caregiving assistance:

- What are the specific care needs? Are they temporary or permanent?
- Can they be met by family or friends who live close by?
- Are the patient's social, spiritual and emotional needs being met?
- Is returning to independent living a treatment goal?
- Are there one or more chronic medical conditions that will intensify over time?
- Is the patient capable of managing necessary medical equipment or medications?
- Can modifications be made to the home?
- Would monitoring services or devices make independent living possible?
- Are health insurance or long-term care insurance benefits available?
- Are there local resources for meals, social activities and transportation?
- Is it time to get on waiting lists for needed services or housing?
- Are there financial resources available for companion or home health services?

If a caregiver will be with the patient for extended periods of time and/or will accompany the patient to provider appointments, the patient's **Good-To-Meet-You- &-In-Case-of-Emergency Profile** will come in handy. It covers emergency and proxy contacts, provider information, medications, allergies and medical history. Have copies available to take along to any new providers, care facilities, urgent care clinics or the hospital (see Chapter Fifteen for specifics on creating this profile).

Keep in mind that there is stiff competition for the services of competent, compassionate caregivers. Do whatever it takes to get ahead of anticipated needs.

You may be the caregiver

If you are responsible for the care of another person, please seek help when you need it—even before you need it. There are many general caregiving resources available, as well as support that addresses the unique needs of persons with specific medical conditions:

- To access a vast collection of caregiver resources: www.caregiverslibrary.org.
- To find ratings for potential third-party care providers: www.medicare.gov - Find

& Compare Providers and http://www.eldercare.gov - Find Help in Your Community.

- To learn about Medicare benefits for specific chronic medical conditions - https://www.medicare.gov - Special Needs Plans.

Addressing your own mental, emotional, spiritual and physical needs as a caregiver will allow you to remain available and able to serve for as long as possible. That may mean attending a support group, getting respite care for your patient, having others fill in briefly while you have a daycation—whatever it takes: https://www.caregiver.org - Taking Care of Yourself. When others offer their help, accept it—and don't be too proud to ask if they don't. Have a backup plan in case you are ever incapacitated yourself on a temporary or permanent basis. [Note that a caregiver does not have medical decision making authority without first being legally recognized as a proxy or guardian.]

There's a reason the flight attendant says, *"If you're responsible for another person, put your own oxygen mask on first."*

You may be the one being cared for

You get no argument from me: Aging or having a temporary or chronic medical condition that leaves you asking for help sucks. Nevertheless, my advice is *Don't be a mule.* I can't even tell you how many times I have personally witnessed or been told about people who refused to have the minimal lifestyle adjustments needed to be safe in their homes. As a result, they were injured and ultimately lost all independence.

Down the road, it may be the diagnosis of a life-limiting or chronic condition or simply "nature's beautiful pageant" that will diminish your ability to care for yourself without some assistance. As soon as possible, start making plans for that day.

- Be honest about your capabilities and limitations.
- When you are blessed to have someone offer help, accept it.
- Do whatever it takes to make the most of your life.

Sometimes asking for help
is the most meaningful example of self-reliance.
Anonymous

CHAPTER NINE

Preventive care

Do you discuss preventive care at your annual checkup or wellness visit? Maybe I should first ask if you're among the 92 percent of American adults who think it's important to see the doctor at least once a year—but also part of the 38 percent who don't get around to it.[26] An annual checkup or wellness visit consists of a physical examination and routine tests such as blood pressure and a full blood panel (tests measuring the glucose level, electrolytes, kidney function, liver function and cholesterol). The goal is to address any patient concerns, to identify potential or developing health care issues and to establish baseline numbers to more easily identify a future variance.

I can argue for or against the annual checkup as a diagnostic tool. Admittedly, there is not a lot of solid research confirming its value in spotting otherwise undetected health care issues. The Medicare Annual Wellness Visit certainly isn't the same physical I got through private health insurance prior to my Happy 65th Birthday. As I discovered, some blood tests are covered by Medicare only every five years unless known issues merit monitoring. But there is something you definitely get with *every* annual wellness exam: An opportunity to be face-to-face with your primary care provider and to share what's going on in your life. Even if you have chronic health conditions and see specialists on a regular basis, an annual physical is the chance to directly communicate with the captain of your health care team.

Preventive care

Preventive care includes tests or procedures meant to either stop a medical condition from occurring or to discover an otherwise hidden health care issue. Although we usually think about regular testing and procedures as being for adults, preventive care is a lifelong pursuit. For a comprehensive list of recommended tests for those under 18, visit this website run by the U.S. Centers for Medicare and Medicaid: www.healthcare.gov - Preventive Care for Children.

As with any proposed medical procedure, you should practice due diligence to determine the unique needs of a particular patient. Here are the most common tests and procedures suggested throughout life:

- Vaccinations, e.g., for childhood diseases, tetanus, influenza, HPV, pneumonia, meningitis, hepatitis (www.cdc.gov - Adult Immunization Chart)
- Mammograms for breast cancer
- Colonoscopies for colorectal cancer
- PSA (prostate-specific antigen) test for prostate cancer
- Eye exams for glaucoma and macular degeneration
- Mental health and substance abuse screenings
- Bone density screening for osteoporosis
- Pelvic examination and pap test for uterine and cervical cancers
- Blood glucose test for diabetes.

Preventive tests or procedures may not be done during a wellness visit because not all are conducted every year and/or some may happen at a facility separate from your primary care provider. If you don't receive reminders for preventive tests, take responsibility to find reliable recommendations for a person of your age, gender and family history. Once you've decided on what and when, put ticklers on your calendar (most online calendars have repeating functions that can be set years in advance).

There are countless sources of preventive care charts and lists (just Google *"preventive care charts,"* if you don't believe me). The U.S. National Library of Medicine has a list of preventive screening procedures by age and gender (https://medlineplus.gov – Health Screening):

- Health screening - men - 18 to 39
- Health screening - men - 40 to 64
- Health screening - men - 65 and older
- Health screening - women - 18 to 39
- Health screening - women - 40 to 64
- Health screening - women - 65 and older

Two more user-friendly and reliable sources are The Centers for Disease Control (www.cdc.gov - CDC Prevention Checklist) and Johns Hopkins Medicine (www.hopkinsmedicine.org - Screening Tests for Common Diseases). For Medicare patients, here are lists and explanations of the preventive procedures covered by Medicare and how often: www.medicare.gov - Medicare coverage for preventive care and www.medicare.gov - Your Guide to Medicare's Preventive Services booklet (or call 1/800-633-4227).

If your family's history includes a specific medical condition, you may want to visit that disease website for targeted preventive care suggestions, such as the

American Cancer Society: www.cancer.org - Cancer Screening Guidelines or the American Heart Association: www.heart.org - Heart Condition Screening. Health care authorities vary in their opinions, so ask your primary care provider for recommendations as well.

Preparing for your annual physical

There's not a lot of prepping to be done for an annual physical, unless you are instructed to fast before blood work. If your health insurance allows, you can have lab work done a day or so ahead of your visit so the results will be available for discussion when you meet with your provider. Personally, I like to get all this stuff over and done with, so I schedule tests such as a mammogram just prior to an annual examination so my provider has my results when we get together. If your primary care provider cannot access results from the testing laboratory, ask that reports be transmitted to him once available. When health insurance does not cover a full blood panel, which your provider's staff can probably tell you, ask if it's advisable for you to have the test. If so, and you can afford it, have it done.

Preparing for any medical test

Another finding in those studies on health literacy was that only 12 percent of American adults understand the instructions needed to prepare for a medical test.[27] Hey, we've all seen the handouts and we empathize. Nevertheless, if you're going to the effort, inconvenience, cost and maybe even pain of having a test, it makes sense to shoot for the most accurate results possible.

Read the instructions and if you don't understand exactly what you are supposed to do—and *not* do—ask questions until it's clear. Talk to friends who have had the same test, like me: over the past 15 years, I've perfected a method of preparing for a colonoscopy that makes the preceding evening a lot more tolerable. Really.

Interpreting test results

I used to have a primary care physician who was scrupulous about mailing a copy of my annual blood panel results to me. I also scrupulously kept them in a file so I could compare the numbers the following year. To this day, I cannot tell you why. Talk about a fool's errand—I didn't have a clue what any of those numbers meant.

These are steps—in order of preference—that you can take once results are available for any diagnostic test you have:

1. You meet with the health care provider to review the results and to hear any recommendations for treatment (good old shared decision making).

2. You get on the phone with the provider and ask to speak to someone who can explain what the test results mean and if there is a next step to be taken.

3. You review the explanatory notes you receive along with the results to be aware of any issues of concern and what, if any, remedial steps need to be taken.

4. You get on the Internet and do your own research on what the numbers mean—in general. Then you arrange to discuss with your provider what *your* numbers mean for *you.*

It is not a coincidence that every one of those steps begins with the word "you."

CHAPTER TEN

Medication

We've grown accustomed to getting a pill for nearly every ailment, to the tune of over four billion prescriptions being filled in America each year.[28] You know, if a little is good, a lot is better. Only now are we beginning to comprehend the potential harm of overprescribing, on oh so many levels. In fact, there is a mushrooming subspecialty of pharmacology called "deprescribing," which means reducing, tapering off or stopping a medication.

The genie is out of the bottle, along with all those pills. It's time to acknowledge that drug literacy is an essential element of health literacy.

Being an informed drug therapy patient

Anytime your provider suggests a new prescription, fully discuss its potential impact on all segments of your life. These questions are based on a guide for that patient-provider conversation from the National Institutes of Health (https://medlineplus.gov - What to Ask Your Doctor):

- What is the name of the drug?
- Why are you prescribing it?
- What is the name of the condition it's intended to treat? (Write it down.)
- Is there a less expensive generic form of the medicine?
- Will I know if it is working and how long will that take?
- How should I store the medicine?
- Is there any potential harmful interaction with drugs I already take?
- How should it be taken?
  - When and how often should I take it? As needed, or on a schedule?
  - Do I take the medicine before, with, or between meals?
  - Are there other medicines or activities I should avoid when taking this medicine?
  - Are there any foods that I should now avoid?
  - Can I drink alcohol when taking this medicine? How much?
- How long will I need to take this prescription?

- What are the potential short-term and long-term side effects of this medicine?
- Will we need to check the medicine's level or any side effects with lab tests?
- If I forget to take a dose, what should I do?
- If I want to quit taking it, is it safe to just stop?[29]

Once you have those answers, choose whether to consent to drug therapy as you would any other medical care. In consultation with your provider, answer the question, *"Considering my personal and treatment goals, is this the right thing for me to do?"*

"Exactly how many pills do you take, anyway?"

Whether you're familiar with the term, you're probably familiar with the concept of *polypharmacy*. It's the use of five or more medications for one or more medical conditions at the same time, and that includes prescriptions, over-the-counter meds, vitamins and herbal supplements. Aging Americans are most likely to suffer the unintended harmful consequences of polypharmacy, which can include frailty, falls, dementia-like symptoms, depression and loss of independence. This predisposition results from the effects of aging on metabolism, brain function and pharmaceuticals (*pharmacodynamics* and *pharmacokinetics*). That and the fact that those between 65 and 84 use an average of 14 to 18 different prescriptions in a year's time.[30] Admittedly, the health care industry's recent angst over polypharmacy is also partly about the money: The practical cost of medication-related health care treatment in America is estimated at $200 billion per annum.

If you or a loved one take five or more medications—especially if taken over a long period of time for multiple conditions or prescribed by more than one provider— you may be overdue for a *Brown Bag Checkup*. It is also referred to as a *Drug Regimen Review* and Medicare calls it a *Medication Therapy Management Program* (a Part D benefit). The *brown bag* reference is because that's an easy way to tote all those bottles to your pharmacist or primary care provider for a comprehensive review—and toss in the over-the-counter meds, vitamins and herbal supplements while you're at it.

Take along the medication records in your **Good-To-Meet-You-&-In-Case-of-Emergency Profile** and be thinking about these issues: Do you address any side affects with another drug remedy or make a lifestyle adjustment? How are medications stored? Is there a reliable system to encourage compliance? Are dosages ever intentionally skipped? If so, why? Please be forthright about how and when each medication is taken and its use, nonuse or inconsistent use. Trust that the provider conducting the evaluation is there to help—not shame—the patient, so aim for complete honesty.

The provider will assess proper use, potential drug-drug, drug-food and drug-disease interactions, duplications, drugs used to counter the side effects of other drugs, nonmedication alternatives and whether prescriptions correspond to current diagnoses. In consultation between the pharmacist and all prescribers, the risks and side effects of each medication can be weighed against its potential benefits as part of the patient's overall treatment plan. What remains are the drugs that work well together for the good of the patient. The final step is for the physician or pharmacist to review all remaining and/or new medications with the patient or caregiver to make sure the purpose and proper use of each is fully understood going forward.

Keeping a record of what, why, when and how

A record of all medications is a vital element of the **Good-To-Meet-You-&-In-Case-of-Emergency Profile** and it's important to keep it updated with changes as time goes on. Your health care providers and/or pharmacist can give you a printed list of your current prescriptions. You may need your provider's assistance to add accurate information about the medical condition each prescription is for, then make your own notes on when and how you take each dosage. Keep printed copies of the **Good-To-Meet-You-&-In-Case-of-Emergency Profile** and/or use an online website or smartphone app to make the information available anytime you:
- Visit a health care provider for the first time.
- Change pharmacists.
- Go to a walk-in or urgent care clinic or emergency room.
- Have an outpatient procedure done or are hospitalized.
- Reside in a rehabilitation center or care facility.
- Are visited by a home health care provider.

Offering an up-to-date copy of medication records will make all providers aware of potentially harmful interactions or duplications before they recommend an additional prescription or medical procedure.

Staying on track with the right tools and system in place

Whether or not your current drug therapy qualifies as polypharmacy, here are some suggestions for giving it the respect it deserves going forward:
- Keep your list of medications current with any additions or changes.
- Use only one pharmacy to fill all prescriptions so potential interactions can be easily detected and avoided.
- Do not share or borrow other people's prescriptions and properly dispose of any medications once expired or no longer being used, for whatever reason.

- Ask if your pharmacist has an automatic refill program and whether it would be an appropriate medication management tool for you or a loved one.
- Always read and understand label instructions and be aware of possible side effects and interactions before taking a medication—prescribed or over-the-counter.
- As part of every annual checkup or wellness exam, include a thorough review of all medications with the primary care provider.
- Don't leave the pharmacy with a new prescription without reviewing dosage instructions and potential side effects with the pharmacist or pharmacy technician.
- Dispensing devices on the market are too numerous to name, except to say that they range from simple $2.99 *Sunday-Saturday* pill minder boxes to electronic dosing machines and smartphone alarm apps. Many pharmacies now dispense in dosage blister packs at no extra charge, so ask. Your pharmacist, provider or an occupational therapist can recommend an appropriate aid for your situation, a system that encourages compliance and the proper storage and dispensing of medications.
- For special circumstances, such as a temporary pain relief prescription or antibiotic, adopt a reliable chart to write down when and what dosages are taken. This is especially important if there are multiple caregivers attending the patient or the patient is self-dosing.

We are just beginning to recognize the importance of health literacy when it comes to drug therapy. Medication literacy is a crucial element of any commitment to be an informed medical decision maker.

CHAPTER ELEVEN

✹

Urgent care and emergency care

You may have noticed an addition to your primary care provider's menu of services over the past few years: an urgent care center. Usually open seven days a week and weekday evenings, it's the stopgap between an appointments-only clinic and the emergency room. In order to respond accordingly, you'll need to recognize the difference between urgent care and emergency care.

Urgent care is for a medical issue that requires attention as soon as possible, but is not serious enough for medical crisis or trauma services. Urgent care patients are typically ambulatory and able to walk into the clinic, rather than being carried in. The flu, an earache and a sprained ankle are good examples of urgent care maladies. Urgent care providers often act as frontline triage experts and may refer the patient on to a specialist or even the emergency room.

Emergency care is for a traumatic injury or medical condition requiring immediate and full-scale attention, such as severe pain, a car accident, head injury or sudden difficulty in speaking or breathing. Emergency departments are usually attached to a hospital. For a medical emergency, time is of the essence and you should err on the side of caution. When in doubt, dial 9-1-1.

Here's a great guide from Mount Sanai Hospital listing typical urgent care and emergency care needs: www.mountsinai.org - Urgent vs. Emergency Care. Now would be a good time to read it and get a better sense of the distinctions.

Being prepared for the unforeseen

Planning for the unexpected is why the questions in Chapter Six should be asked well ahead of a health care crisis. Knowing in advance your alternatives for after-hours, urgent care and emergency needs saves valuable time. That same proactive attitude of yours is why I know you will already have the **Good-To-Meet-You-&-In-Case-of-Emergency Profile** in print or available on a smartphone app to take along in the event of urgent or emergency care.

For *urgent care matters*, your primary care provider may keep appointments open each day or you may be able to see an associate, nurse practitioner or physician's assistant in the practice. Check to see what options are available with your own provider before you head to the walk-in or urgent care clinic to be seen by a stranger.

For *emergencies*, first you call 9-1-1, tell the dispatcher about the person's symptoms or injury as calmly as possible and then do as the dispatcher instructs while you wait to be transported by emergency personnel.

Emergencies: getting there and being there

How your primary care physician or specialist prefers to handle the hospitalization of a patient—including emergencies—is information to have ahead of time.

- What hospital is the provider affiliated with?
- Does the provider use a hospitalist to attend to his patients? If so, who is it?
- How is primary care provider-hospitalist communication handled?

If there is the opportunity to choose a hospital at the time of the emergency—which depends on the location and nature of the crisis—you can direct emergency personnel to that facility. These are my recommendations for reacting in an emergency:

1. Call 9-1-1. Do <u>not</u> attempt to transport someone with symptoms that may possibly be life-threatening. Yes, it could be embarrassing to travel by ambulance for what turns out to be only a panic attack. However, it beats dying in route to the hospital because the friend who's driving you there doesn't know CPR. And is busy driving.

2. If you are with the patient when emergency personnel arrive, calmly relate the nature of the injury or symptoms. If the patient is unable to speak, offer relevant information such as the patient's age and usual level of cognitive function and mobility. Include chronic conditions and any recent illnesses or procedures. Offer the **Good-To-Meet-You-&-In-Case-of-Emergency Profile**. After all, you are now the patient's voice.

3. If you receive the call that a loved one has been taken to the emergency room and you can safely get there, go. If you drive, concentrate on being safe—text and make phone calls to other concerned friends or family once you arrive. Not sure you should drive yourself? Then arrange for transportation.

4. When you get to the hospital, call the patient's primary care provider to tell him where you are. Verify that the provider will be attending the patient or get the name and contact information for the appropriate specialist or hospitalist recommended by the primary care provider.

5. Notify the patient's emergency contact and health care proxy, if they are persons other than you.

6. If a specialist or hospitalist will be the patient's attending physician while in the hospital, contact that provider and let them know you and the patient are in the emergency department.

7. Make the patient's **Good-To-Meet-You-&-In-Case-of-Emergency Profile** available to hospital personnel and provide the name and contact information for the patient's attending physician (the primary care provider, specialist or hospitalist who will be overseeing the patient's care while hospitalized).

8. Let the emergency personnel know that the patient's attending physician is awaiting an update on the patient's condition once the patient has been stabilized.

9. Determine which person on the emergency room team will be communicating with you and with the patient's attending physician.

Note: *A Health Care Advance Directive is not a medical order, so unless a patient has an Out-of-hospital Do-not-resuscitate order (OOH-DNR) or an equivalent POLST-type medical order, emergency medical personnel are required by law to attempt to save and/or revive a patient.*

Here is a practical communication tool from Dr. Ferdinando L. Mirarchi. His checklist is meant for medical professionals evaluating a patient who is critically ill or an emergency patient who may require cardiopulmonary resuscitation (CPR). I think it also serves as valuable guidance for patients and advocates.

The goal is to determine whether the patient's advance directives—expressed verbally or in writing—are known and then incorporated into the patient's treatment plan. Called *The Resuscitation Pause* or *Advance Directive Pause,* it utilizes Dr. Mirarchi's *ABCDE's of the Living Will*:

A. Ask the patient or health care proxy to be clear about the patient's intentions as expressed in any existing Health Care Advance Directive.

B. Be clear about whether this emergency is a triggering event for the use of life prolonging measures *or* a treatable critical or emergency condition.

C. Communicate clearly whether the condition is reversible and treatable and if the prognosis is good or poor.

D. Design and discuss a plan of care with specific next steps and who will take those steps.

E. Explain that it is okay to withhold or withdraw life sustaining treatment, and if it is the appropriate next step, explain and arrange for palliative and/or hospice care for the patient.[31]

The time to repair the roof is when the sun is shining.
John Fitzgerald Kennedy

CHAPTER TWELVE

ॐ☙

Facing a critical decision

Few words are more transformative than "Your tests came back and I have some bad news." A friend's husband describes the moments just after learning he had cancer: "I don't recall anything the doctor said that day. I was too busy listening to the voice in my head, '*You're going to die. You're going to die.*'"

Whether you're facing an unforeseen diagnosis or surgery, a recommendation for invasive diagnostic tests or even an elective procedure, you have important, potentially life-altering options to consider. Complex medical conditions merit complex decision making, so think of this as Part III of Chapter Seven's shared decision making on steroids. Whether you are advocating for yourself or for another, the choices you make must be *fully informed* choices.

Gathering information

If tests are needed to identify a medical condition or to confirm a diagnosis, start by getting the answers to these questions:
- What is the purpose of these tests?
- How accurate are these tests and what do we hope to learn from the results?
- Are there any risks in having the tests?
- Will I need any follow-up or repeat tests in the future?

Your provider may need to seek counsel from a specialist before beginning the shared decision making process with you. Once all information needed to discuss the issue is available, you should meet face-to-face to learn about your diagnosis and your options for care. Keep in mind that some questions will be irrelevant and can be skipped, depending on the specific health issue:
- What is the name of the disease or medical condition? (Write it down.)
- Do you have a brochure or website you can refer me to for more information?
- Do we know what caused this?
- What is the likely prognosis, in the near future and down the road?
- Do I need to be careful about infecting others with this disease?

- Are there any activities I need to avoid right now because of this condition?
- What short-term and long-term symptoms can I expect and should I watch for?
- Will my needs for caregiving change as the condition progresses?
- Are there home modifications or special medical equipment I will need?
- Is this disease curable?
- If there is no cure, what is likely to happen over the course of time?
- As we discuss available treatment options, is the surgery, procedure or drug therapy:
  - An attempt to cure the medical condition or disease.
  - To treat symptoms, without intending to cure the disease.
  - To provide palliative or comfort care.
  - To prolong my life without an intent to treat the disease.
- For each treatment option, what are the potential side effects?
- Is palliative care an option for any discomfort or painful side effects?
- How will we know if the treatment is effective?
- What risks and benefits come with each treatment option?
- Is there research on the probability of success for these treatments?
- Are the treatments readily available?
- What are the costs of the treatments?
- If needed, are there any financial aid programs available to cover treatment costs?
- What is likely to happen if I decide to have no curative treatment or I delay it?
- What if I start the treatment and then decide to stop?
- Will I need to be hospitalized now or at some point in the future?
- If there is a surgery, how long will it take me to recover?
- How will my lifestyle or work life be affected during these treatments?
- Will I need home assistance or rehabilitation during or after treatment?
- Do I qualify for any alternative treatments, such as experimental or clinical trials?
- What treatment plan do you recommend?
- How soon do I need to make a decision?

There are three key elements in making a medical decision with potential long-term or life-limiting consequences: information, information and information.

Getting a second opinion

If visiting the doctor brings on anxiety, you are not alone. There's even a name for it: *White coat syndrome* or *white coat hypertension* causes a spike in blood pressure from the fear of, well, having one's blood pressure taken. So, suggesting that your provider is mistaken about your diagnosis sounds like even more fun, eh? Rest assured, a health care professional who has your best interests in mind will not be offended. You should consider a second opinion:

- If the treatment options or side effects have serious or life-threatening risks.
- If there is a question about the certainty of the diagnosis.
- If the treatment is experimental in nature.
- If your health insurer requires a second opinion.
- If you keep getting that funny feeling in the back of your head.

Do independent research and ask friends or other health care professionals not directly associated with the first provider to recommend another specialist. Ask for your medical records to be copied to the second provider and think ahead (making notes) of questions you have. Based on the second opinion, you should be equipped to make an informed choice. You may even ask them to consult with each other and devise a treatment plan that incorporates both perspectives, keeping your priorities and best interests in mind.

This is *your life* we're talking about. Be your own best advocate.

Understanding probabilities

Media stories about health care often feature eye-catching headlines on the extraordinary success of a new drug or lifestyle change. Along your health care journey, you may hear similar probabilities about a medical condition and/or treatment option so it's crucial that you understand what they really mean (and don't freak out if you hear the term *morbidity*; it's just another word for *disease*).

[These are fictitious statistics for illustration only.] *Absolute risk* is the chance of getting a disease over a specified time period: 20 percent of smokers have an absolute risk of getting lung cancer in their lives. *Relative risk* is the chance of getting a disease compared to a person in another group: Compared to a nonsmoker with a 2 percent chance of getting lung cancer, a smoker's relative risk is 10 times as high.

If you compare the absolute risk of a smoker getting lung cancer (20 percent) to the absolute risk for a nonsmoker (2 percent), you see that not smoking causes an *absolute risk reduction* of 18 percent. That makes sense. But what we usually see in the headlines is the *relative risk reduction:* "Being a nonsmoker will reduce your risk of getting lung cancer by 90 percent," because a nonsmoker's 2 percent risk is 90 percent less than a smoker's 20 percent risk.

See how that works? Words matter. The potential significance of this distinction is obvious if you are comparing treatment options. *Example*: Research shows that in a group of 2,000 people receiving no treatment for a disease, 20 will die within two years (a 1 percent chance of dying). For the group receiving treatment, only 10 people die within two years (a .5 percent chance). That's an *absolute risk reduction* of one-half of one percent (1.0 percent minus .5 percent) but a *relative risk reduction* of *50 percent* (.5 percent is half of 1.0 percent). A 50 percent reduction in risk sounds pretty good, but maybe not as impressive when you consider that it's just 10 fewer deaths in a group of 2,000 people. If you also learn that every participant who received treatment suffered debilitating side effects, it becomes even less persuasive.

From a second study, the risk of dying without the treatment is 20 in 50—rather than 2,000—while the risk with treatment is 10 in 50. The *relative risk reduction* is the same 50 percent (10 is 50 percent of 20), but now the *absolute risk reduction* is 20 percent (40 percent minus 20 percent), rather than .5 percent and that's 10 people out of only 50. You may decide it's worth enduring the harmful side effects.[32]

I know, it makes my head hurt, too, but this is what the process of evaluating risks versus benefits is about: not just getting data but putting it into perspective with relevant details and truly understanding its meaning to you. Remember that probabilities are just that, the odds of an outcome—not a guaranty. Read the fine print on the chances for success and potential side effects of a lifestyle change, preventive drug therapy or disease treatment. That's the only way to make an informed decision and choose the best option for you.

The prerogative to change your mind

Informed consent means voluntarily agreeing to, refusing to agree to or requesting the withdrawal of a medical procedure with full understanding of the foreseeable risks, benefits, possible alternatives, uncertainties and the option of having no treatment. Because you have the right to first consent before undergoing any medical treatment, you also have the right to *withdraw* consent. In other words, you can agree to a treatment plan and then change your mind later. Yes, there may be irreversible consequences from having begun treatment and/or foregoing another available option, but that reinforces the importance of being fully informed up front.

It's my inner lawyer talking now . . .

What can I say, I'm an attorney, so I can't *not* talk to you about the legal issues raised by a life-limiting diagnosis. If a health care provider says you have a medical condition that may shorten your life or may gradually diminish your decision making capacity, the time to plan ahead for either eventuality is *as soon as possible*.

Concerning future health care decisions, work through the process of considering, communicating and documenting your instructions with Health Care Advance Directives while you still have the indisputable capacity to do so. That will ease your own burden as you continue to self-manage care as well as reduce your proxy's worries in the future, if substitute decision making is needed. In case you are now the caregiver for another person, make plans for their wellbeing if you are not able to continue in that role down the road.

The same goes for financial assets and any property you own. Consult immediately with a competent elder law or estate attorney who is experienced in the preservation and uninterrupted management of assets in the event of future incapacity. For example, a Durable Power of Attorney for Financial Matters can be executed by anyone with legal competence. However, once decision making capacity comes into question, creating that document is no longer an option and the only way to access or convey assets will be through the expense, time and legal process of a conservatorship (in some states, "guardianship" refers to both asset management *and* oversight of the person). Issues to consider include locating all assets; reviewing how title is held on real estate, bank and brokerage accounts and vehicles; estate planning; online account passwords; a business succession plan; employee sick leave, family leave, disability or retirement benefits; a strategy for asset preservation in case of future Medicaid dependency; and the practical considerations of remaining in or disposing of primary and second homes.

Making a record of advance directives for substitute decision making and the use of life prolonging measures can relieve stress for the patient and enables future caregivers to honor known wishes for care. Taking care of business matters while you still can not only preserves assets, it also conserves the patient's and loved ones' energy and resources for dealing with what may come.

CHAPTER THIRTEEN

৯০ ০৩

Palliative care

Not quite sure what *palliative care* is all about? You're not alone. Most folks think it has something to do with dying and that's half right. Unless you understand the full meaning of palliative care and the crucial role it can play in a treatment plan, you may miss life-changing opportunities to incorporate it for yourself or a loved one. Let's start by correctly defining the term.

Palliative care focuses on improving a patient's quality of life by addressing the relief of serious disease symptoms without an intent to treat the medical condition. It is also used to alleviate the adverse side effects of therapy, such as radiation or a surgical procedure. Palliative care is given *in addition* to treatment for the underlying disease and is appropriate anytime a patient has comfort needs. We associate palliative care with end of life because palliative care is, indeed, the foundation of hospice care, but that is not its only role. Simply put: all hospice care is palliative but not all palliative care is hospice. Because the introduction of palliative care is based on patient *need*—rather than diagnosis or prognosis—there is no prerequisite that the patient be approaching the end of life or even that the patient's medical condition is life-limiting.

There are palliative care doctors and there are also interdisciplinary palliative care teams that may include a physician; a pharmacist; a physical, massage or occupational therapist; a social worker; a psychiatrist or psychologist; a nutritionist; religious or spiritual counselors; and trained volunteers. While the palliative care provider or team focuses on the patient's comfort and quality of life, the disease specialist can give full attention to treating the primary medical condition or disorder. For example:

• The cardiologist deals with the patient's congestive heart failure and the palliative care specialist addresses symptoms such as shortness of breath and edema.

• The oncologist oversees the cancer patient's chemotherapy and radiation treatments while palliative care addresses painful symptoms and the treatment's side effects of nausea, fatigue, anxiety and depression.

• The pulmonologist treats the patient's COPD, leaving the palliative care team to address breathlessness and to help the patient and family make necessary decisions about the patient's lifestyle and living arrangements.

Although it is not the primary goal of palliative care to treat the patient's disease, we now know that addressing the emotional, social, spiritual and physical elements of "total pain" can directly impact a patient's willingness to stick with a treatment plan and even the ability to heal. Palliative care includes traditional pain relief as well as holistic treatments such as massage, guided imagery and talk therapy. It may also embrace the patient's immediate network of family members or friends by guiding difficult decision making and coordinating treatment plan logistics.

Patients and loved ones sometimes resist the introduction of palliative care. That can happen if its function is not properly explained and they wrongly assume the medical team has abandoned all treatment in favor of hospice. Poor communication can result in a lost opportunity, because not only can palliative care be complementary to the treatment of any serious disease, many studies have verified that the early introduction of palliative care in the treatment of cancer:

- Improves symptoms, health care-related quality of life and the patient's mood.
- Aids in the decision making process.
- Reduces the use of aggressive medical care at the end of life.
- Improves family and patient satisfaction.[33]

The most remarkable finding to date? That lung cancer patients who began palliative care at the time of diagnosis survived 25 percent longer than those for whom palliative care was delayed.[34]

For a comprehensive review of the role that palliative care can play in the treatment of 26 major diseases, visit this site: https://getpalliativecare.org - Palliative Care for Disease Types. You will also find that websites for most specific medical conditions now also address the uses and advantages of palliative care. One example is www.cancer.gov - Palliative Care in Cancer.

If palliative care is suggested for you or a loved one, ask questions until you fully understand its intended use and the reason behind the recommendation. If you or someone you are caring for is suffering with the symptoms of a medical condition or the side effects of therapy, inquire about including palliative care in the treatment plan. Although it may be more difficult to access those services outside a hospital setting, don't give up. Actively counsel with your health care providers to fully address all aspects of patient care, including comfort and making the most out of life, whether measured in days or decades.

CHAPTER FOURTEEN

As the end of life approaches

Is it the curative treatment for a middle-aged cancer patient that is failing? A young person with an irreversible brain injury? Or diminishing symptom control for a 93-year-old with congestive heart failure? No matter the patient's age or diagnosis as the end of life approaches, the right to informed consent never lapses, even though it may need to be exercised by a proxy on behalf of the patient. As long as the patient is alive, patient autonomy endures. In fact, end of life is the last—and sometimes the most significant—opportunity to recognize and honor the patient's unique values, preferences and priorities. And there are no do-overs when it comes to dying, so it's imperative that we get it right the first time.

Medical futility means a treatment or procedure is unlikely to produce any beneficial results for the patient. Predicting medical futility can be challenging, even heartbreaking, and is sometimes based only on a provider's best guess. Few decisions are more daunting for health care professionals and loved ones than choosing when to remain hopeful for a positive outcome and when to acknowledge that it is in the patient's best interest to focus solely on palliative care. It is not possible or medically acceptable to offer everything to everyone who requests it. Instead, we wrestle to balance the patient's condition and priorities with the provider's ethical obligations, the wishes of loved ones and the meshing gears of the health care system.

Accurately predicting the progression and duration of a disease is complex and subject to unforeseeable variables. That's when open and honest communication through shared decision making is crucial to maintaining patient autonomy. It may seem too simple to be true, but the best way to learn what another person is thinking is to *ask*. When a patient with a terminal condition wants an answer to the question, "*What now?*," Dr. Atul Gawande, author of *Being Mortal*, relies on these questions to best determine the patient's priorities and to design a course of treatment that respects the patient's autonomy:

1. What is your understanding of where you are with your condition or your illness at this time?
2. What are your fears and worries for the future?

3. What are your goals if time is short?
4. What outcomes would be unacceptable to you?[35]

Being aware of and acknowledging the purpose for each medical treatment along the trajectory of the disease—is it meant to cure, treat, comfort or prolong life—allows patient and providers to adjust the treatment plan as circumstances dictate. The end of life is no time to abandon the goal of respecting patient autonomy. Everyone must be willing to ask the most difficult of questions and adapt to an ever-changing definition of "a good day" for the patient, because what they say is true: *"Once you've seen one dying patient, you've seen one dying patient."*

For loved ones, caregivers and even health care professionals, choosing to decline measures meant to prolong life may seem disloyal to the patient. However, providers who understand that no longer treating the disease does *not* mean no longer treating the patient are best equipped to facilitate the acceptance of life's inevitable end. The late doctor and gifted author of *When breath becomes air*, Paul Kalanithi, acknowledged soon after his stage IV lung cancer diagnosis that *"My relationship with statistics changed as soon as I became one."*[36]

Hospice care

Hospice is an interdisciplinary approach to patient care when the primary or attending provider certifies that life expectancy is six months or less (the standard for Medicare and most health insurers). The goal for a hospice patient's treatment plan is to help the patient live as well as possible—as defined by the patient directly or through his proxy—until natural death comes. Hospice care focuses on the dying patient's overall quality of life and comfort, so further treatment of the terminal illness is discontinued and the focus is on managing symptoms of the disease and of the dying process through palliative care.

Suffering should not be accepted as a natural and inevitable part of the dying process—it is not. Along with comfort care addressing physical symptoms and pain management, hospice includes spiritual, social and emotional support for the patient. Unlike most other health care disciplines, hospice care encompasses the welfare of the patient's loved ones, including bereavement services after the patient has passed. The therapies of holistic hospice care may include pain relief; massage; physical, speech and occupational therapies; meditation; pastoral and bereavement counseling; and complementary care such as art, aroma, music, pet, Reiki and healing touch therapies.

Hospice care can make it possible for the patient's closest family members and friends to turn from being full-time caregivers to focusing on spending quality time with the patient, however long that may be. The Medicare hospice benefit also covers respite care, which provides short-term residential hospice care to address an acute palliative care challenge or to temporarily relieve the usual caregiver.

Consistently when surveyed, 80 percent of Americans would prefer to die at home,[37] which, coincidentally, is the same percentage of those who don't manage to do so.[38] Twenty-nine percent of all deaths occur in a hospital;[39] for hospice patients, however, that number is only nine percent.[40] That says it all: hospice is about considering and respecting the patient's personal priorities until life comes to its natural end.

Understanding options for end-of-life care

If you're a fan of Star Wars, you're familiar with Master Yoda and one of his many astute observations: *"Death is a natural part of life."* You can also imagine that if Yoda were asked about the process of dying, he might say, *"Only when and how. There is no if."* It's the *how* that is worrisome for most folks. Rest assured, when curative measures are no longer a viable option, there are still opportunities to respect patient autonomy with decision making that directly impacts the patient's quality of life, to its very end.

There is no way to achieve effective shared decision making other than having all parties speak the same language. As the end of life approaches, confusion often results from a lack of communication between patient, proxy and provider. Begin by reviewing the Glossary in the back of this book and also recall that it is the role of advance directives to communicate how proxy decision makers should act on behalf of the patient. When it seems there is so little that can be done, the remaining gift for a dying loved one is to honor their wishes for care, whether communicated in written directives or whispered as you hold hands at the bedside.

Some questions should only be answered by the patient: *What parts of life—given the available alternatives—are most important to you? Maintaining dignity and a degree of independence? Not being in pain? Being able to communicate with loved ones? Having enough time to say goodbye? Feeding yourself? Writing a letter to family and friends? Seeking forgiveness or saying "I love you"? Sharing that favorite family recipe one more time? Checking off an item from a Bucket List?*

These are among the matters that should be taken into account when considering a treatment plan for a dying patient:

• Review Health Care Advance Directives to verify the patient's care preferences and the appointment of a proxy, if needed. In the absence of written directives—or any change of heart—ask the patient about wishes for end-of-life treatment and determine who will act as the surrogate decision maker.

• Determine whether the patient qualifies for hospice, whether there is health insurance coverage or other funds available for hospice and whether care will be provided in a hospice residence, the hospital, a care facility or the patient's home.

• Make sure everyone understands the patient's intent when wishes for care are verbalized, such as "*I don't want to be a burden*" or "*Just let me go.*"

• As it is appropriate for the circumstances, discuss the risks and benefits associated with the use of or withholding of life prolonging measures such as a ventilator, a feeding tube or intravenous hydration (use of an IV). Clarify when it may no longer be medically sound to feed the person or to give them liquids.

• Because advance directives are not medical orders, agree on the patient's code status in the event of a respiratory or cardiac crisis. As needed, request medical orders such as a Do-not-resuscitate order, Do-not-hospitalize order or Comfort Care Only order so that providers are properly authorized to act in accordance with directives.

• Review the advisability of discontinuing medications such as blood pressure drugs, statins or antibiotics and the deactivation of medical devices such as a pacemaker or an implantable cardioverter defibrillator (ICD).

• If options are available, discuss where the patient would prefer to die, who should be present at the end of life and environmental preferences (pets, music, reading, touching, praying, being outdoors, etc.).

• Address the patient's and loved ones' questions about the course of the disease, such as *Does there have to be pain at the end of life? Will we know when the patient is about to die? Is it safe to leave the patient's side for a while? Will the patient be able to hear and know we are present? What will death look like?*

• Including the issues of anxiety or fear, constantly assess the patient's level of pain. If full sedation is necessary for relief of uncontrollable pain, ask whether the patient has a preference about being conscious at the time of death.

• Understand clearly what the law allows your health care providers to do as the patient is dying. Except in the six jurisdictions in the United States that permit physician-assisted suicide, it is illegal to intentionally hasten a person's death.

• As difficult as it may be, accept that decisions which honor and embrace the patient's whole being and personal priorities may not prolong the patient's life.

Steps to take when death is imminent

It will ease the survivors' burden and perhaps reduce stress for the dying patient to prepare for matters that demand attention as the end of life approaches and soon after the patient's death. If the patient can communicate, ask who should be made aware of his condition and passing. Gather contact information for family members, closest friends and the patient's attorney and financial advisors. Make sure there is accessibility to account numbers and paperwork for real estate, financial assets, insurance policies, passwords for online accounts, Social Security records, etc. If the patient is responsible for dependents, such as children or elderly parents, take steps for their care (and don't forget the four-legged family members). Any instructions for the disposition of remains and a funeral or memorial ceremony should be readily accessible. As long as the patient has decision making capacity, there may be legal means to simplify the eventual probate process. Consult with a competent estate or elder law attorney, if time allows.

For a patient in hospice care, the provider will guide the process once death has occurred. Family members are usually encouraged to spend as much time as they wish with their loved one and there may be religious or memorial rituals to be performed before the body is removed. No matter where death occurs, as loved ones acknowledge the need to say goodbye to a family member or friend, this is not a time to be rushed. Acknowledging loss is a process.

Leaving a legacy not measured in dollars and cents

When I wrote *Last things first, just in case* in 2006, I included one little chapter on an ancient tradition I had just learned about, Ethical Wills. Readers wanted to know more, and so did I. In 2010, I wrote a book devoted to Ethical Wills and leaving a permanent record of one's beliefs and values, life lessons and hopes for the future.[41] The first Ethical Will is found in the Book of Genesis. Thirty-five hundred years later, this practice continues to impart wisdom, communicate affection and identify the most important parts of one's journey: the impact we have had on the lives of others.

Although I first learned about Ethical Wills when I witnessed dying patients creating them in hospice care, they are not a practice reserved for end of life. An Ethical Will can mark any milestone, such as empty-nesting, retirement, the birth of a grandchild, a family wedding or each new year's beginning. I encourage you to write a letter, make a video, highlight favorite Bible verses or share a collection of meaningful quotations—whatever media is most likely to get you to share the message of what you stand for. It will be a priceless treasure, perhaps for generations to come.

What you leave behind is not what is engraved in stone monuments,
but what is woven into the lives of others.
Pericles

CHAPTER FIFTEEN

❧ ❧

What? There's paperwork, too?

We've come to the third and final building block of health literacy: action steps. Having a health literate brain is our goal, but there is really no reason to store loads of vital statistics in your head. And if your ability to communicate is ever impaired in the future, a written record of personal information can be invaluable. It will assist the health care professionals treating you as well as the loved ones acting as decision makers on your behalf.

Good-To-Meet-You-&-In-Case-of-Emergency Profile

If you have a medical emergency and are unable to communicate, how will first responders access the information they need? And every time you meet a new provider, go to an urgent care clinic or have an outpatient procedure, someone is going to want to know about you. It's time to learn all that needs to be included in your **Good-To-Meet-You-&-In-Case-of-Emergency Profile**. To be sure your relevant history is available—and to assemble all this information just *once*—your profile needs to include:

• Names and contact information for friends or family members to be notified in a medical emergency.

• A list of existing medical conditions, allergies, medications and medical devices.

• Names and contact information of all providers, both primary care and specialists.

• Health insurance information, including any prescription coverage.

• Names and contact information for the health care proxy and alternate proxy.

• The patient's Health Care Advance Directives and any other relevant documents, such as an OOH-DNR, organ donation registration or instructions for final disposition.

Now you get to decide how to make that record.

If you want to go old school—and there's nothing wrong with that because I want you to do whatever you are willing to do—take a few minutes and copy the wallet card in this chapter, print and complete it and keep it next to your driver's license or identification form. And make an extra copy to keep in your fanny pack if you go for walks or bike rides. Do the same with the MEDICATIONS PROFILE and MEDICAL PROFILE forms included here. If you don't like my versions, there's a jillion of those free online, as well. After completion, either scan and upload to a flash drive or make lots of print copies and give them to your emergency contact and proxies; keep a set in your glove compartment; and put one under a magnet on the frig.

There are also many options for online medical recordkeeping. If you use a smartphone, you'll want an app. Most are free for basic data, but even if you're willing to pay for bells and whistles, prices are low. I give a big *thumbs down* to the federal government's *ibluebutton* program. Online use is free but the app is not, and the manual input is a pain. However, I have tried and like https://carezone.com and www.trackmymedicalrecords.com and www.mymedicalapp.com. All are easy to use and allow you to download other documents, such as your advance directives or a printout of your medications. If you wish, you can even scan insurance cards and prescription bottles; some apps can be synchronized with your provider's own online patient portal. Search "consumer medical record apps" and prepare to be dazzled.

Another option is to wear medical record bling. Choose from an assortment of flash drive jewelry, key fobs or teeny tiny memory sticks (perhaps taped to the back of your driver's license?) that will hold your entire medical record, along with emergency information. Google: "medical alert flash drive" to see oodles of choices. Reasonably priced and very cool.

Health Care Advance Directives

A Health Care Advance Directive is a legal document that includes the appointment of a substitute medical decision maker (a Durable Power of Attorney for Health Care) and directives for the use of life-extending and life prolonging measures in case a triggering event occurs (a Living Will). It is now common for these two legal documents to be joined together in a combination advance directive.

Practically speaking, it is impossible to make decisions ahead of time concerning a future, unknown health care situation. Don't misunderstand, I'm a big fan of Advance Care Planning. But I believe its real value is in motivating us to think ahead about our care preferences, choose who should speak for us and provide a process for substitute decision making guidance in *any* health care situation, not just the end of life. A Health Care Advance Directive should ask and answer these two very important questions:

If you are ever too ill to think or speak for yourself,
who do you want to speak for you?

and

When do you think enough is enough?

After years of frustration with outdated and confusing advance directive documents, I created my own version. Nevertheless, it doesn't really matter what form you choose, as long as it accurately reflects your care preferences and lights the path to informed decision making for patient, proxy and physician. Honestly, I'd take a productive conversation about decision making over a poorly drafted advance directive form any day, even knowing there can be unintended consequences from not having a written directive (Chapter Five).

At a minimum, a Health Care Advance Directive should include:
- The appointment of a health care proxy and alternate proxy and authorization for substitute decision making by them.
- The proxy's duties and responsibilities (which also makes it a great guide for the crucial conversation that begins with *"Will you be my proxy?"*).
- A step-by-step process for making decisions in *any* health care situation.
- Clearly communicated wishes for the use of life-extending measures in case a triggering event occurs, such as a terminal condition, irreversible unconsciousness or late stage dementia.

If you want to learn more about Advance Care Planning and end-of-life treatment options, spend 180 minutes reading my book, *The practical guide to Health Care Advance Directives*. It's a worthwhile investment of time if you're aiming for comprehensive health literacy.

Once you've executed your Health Care Advance Directives, make them available to your proxies and loved ones and incorporate them into your **Good-To-Meet-You-&-In-Case-of-Emergency Profile**.

What to do when you're asked to sign something

Unless you happen to be an attorney, it's not reasonable to assume you are fluent in legalese. Repeat after me: *"Could someone please tell me the purpose of this form and what it says in plain language?"* Now, here's the thing: it's safe to say that you will not be permitted to change the terms of a consent form or HIPAA (the Health Insurance Portability and Accountability Act of 1996) form. Refusing to execute them is also not an option. I am only suggesting that you should be clear about what you sign before you sign it. You can ask for a copy of all paperwork prior to a procedure to read it ahead of time. Or here's an idea: take it along into the examination room and ask the doctor to explain it to you. That might prove to be interesting.

Let's just admit we all stopped reading those annoying HIPAA forms sometime in the last millennium. There is, however, something I do want you to verify before you sign off: Make sure privacy forms include the name of anyone who may be making decisions on behalf of the patient so they can be given updates by providers—most especially if there is no appointed proxy and/or an immediate family member available.

If you are signing any form on behalf of someone else as that person's health care proxy or guardian, verify that its terms agree with your understanding of the consent you are granting. Also, do not accept financial responsibility for the patient's care unless that is what you mean to do.

Turning advance directives into medical orders

Because a Health Care Advance Directive is not legally binding in a medical emergency, written and actionable medical orders must be issued that echo the terms of the patient's or decision maker's instructions. For a person who is terminally ill, frail, elderly or has a life-threatening chronic medical condition, there should be a patient-proxy-provider conversation about whether specific orders, such as a Do-not-resuscitate order (DNR) or a POLST (Physician Orders for Life-Sustaining Treatment) order should be executed, well before any medical crisis.

The first step is to have a thorough discussion with the primary care or attending physician about what the order means and what treatment will be given to the patient, with and without the order. It is especially important that everyone—patient, proxy and concerned loved ones—fully understand how health care personnel will respond to medical emergencies such as respiratory or cardiac arrest.

The suitability of these orders depends on the patient's medical condition, long-term treatment plan and personal values, preferences and priorities. Whatever orders are issued should be clearly noted in the patient's record, communicated to all staff and shown on an identifying patient wrist band, as appropriate. As with any informed consent, such orders can be reviewed, amended or withdrawn in the future.

Instructions for funeral or memorial plans

Verify any special requirements in your state's law about instructions for the disposition of a body or memorial rituals. Also check on whether there are statutory restrictions on naming someone to carry out those wishes. Once you are sure of the rules, any arrangements you make ahead of time will ease the burden on your survivors, as well as making sure you get the send-off you want. Make sure any instructions are easily accessible (not in the safety deposit box, where they may not be discovered until weeks after your death). By the way, where is the key to the safety deposit box? And which bank is it at?

Wallet card front:

Name: _____ D.O.B.:_____

Emergency contact: _____

Home phone: _____ Cell phone: _____

Health care proxy: _____

Home phone: _____ Cell phone: _____

Alternate proxy: _____

Home phone: _____ Cell phone: _____

Wallet card back:

Physician: _____ Phone: _____

Hospital affiliation: _____

Medical conditions: _____

_____

Drug allergies: _____

Medical devices: _____

_____

MEDICATIONS PROFILE FOR _____ as of _____

(patient)   (date)

(Include over-the-counter medications, vitamins and any herbal supplements you take.)

Name of the drug: _____ Prescribing provider: _____
This drug was prescribed for (medical condition): _____
Dose: _____ When taken: _____ How taken: _____
Pharmacy where this prescription is filled: _____

(name)   (phone)

Name of the drug: _____ Prescribing provider: _____
This drug was prescribed for (medical condition): _____
Dose: _____ When taken: _____ How taken: _____
Pharmacy where this prescription is filled: _____

(name)   (phone)

Name of the drug: _____ Prescribing provider: _____
This drug was prescribed for (medical condition): _____
Dose: _____ When taken: _____ How taken: _____
Pharmacy where this prescription is filled: _____

(name)   (phone)

Name of the drug: _____ Prescribing provider: _____
This drug was prescribed for (medical condition): _____
Dose: _____ When taken: _____ How taken: _____
Pharmacy where this prescription is filled: _____

(name)   (phone)

Name of the drug: _____ Prescribing provider: _____
This drug was prescribed for (medical condition): _____
Dose: _____ When taken: _____ How taken: _____
Pharmacy where this prescription is filled: _____

(name)   (phone)

Name of the drug: _____ Prescribing provider: _____
This drug was prescribed for (medical condition): _____
Dose: _____ When taken: _____ How taken: _____
Pharmacy where this prescription is filled: _____

(name)   (phone)

Name of the drug: _____ Prescribing provider: _____
This drug was prescribed for (medical condition): _____
Dose: _____ When taken: _____ How taken: _____
Pharmacy where this prescription is filled: _____

(name)   (phone)

MEDICAL PROFILE FOR _____ as of _____
(patient)   (date)

Date of birth: _____ Address: _____

Home phone: _____ Cell phone: _____

Emergency contact: _____ Phone: _____

I have a: ____ **Living Will** ____ **Durable Power of Attorney for Health Care**

Health care proxy: _____ Phone: _____

Alternate health care proxy: _____ Phone: _____

Existing medical conditions: _____
_____
_____

Implanted medical devices: _____

Drug allergy: _____ Known reaction: _____
Drug allergy: _____ Known reaction: _____
Drug allergy: _____ Known reaction: _____
Drug allergy: _____ Known reaction: _____

Other allergy: _____ Known reaction: _____
Other allergy: _____ Known reaction: _____

Primary Health Insurance: _____ Policy No. _____

Address: _____ Phone: _____

Secondary Health Insurance: _____ Policy No. _____

Address: _____ Phone: _____

Prescription Insurance provider: _____ Policy No. _____

Address: _____ Phone: _____

Primary care physician: _____

Address: _____ Phone: _____

Condition being treated: _____

Pharmacy: _____ Phone: _____
Dentist: _____ Phone: _____

Specialist: _____
Address: _____ Phone: _____
Condition being treated: _____

Specialist: _____
Address: _____ Phone: _____
Condition being treated: _____

CLOSING REMARKS

୫୭ଓୠ

Well, there you have it. Now finishing the task of achieving health literacy is up to you.

I kept getting the feeling I had something more to say before we part and then it came to me: *Thank you*, for thinking enough of yourself to invest the time and effort in preserving your rights to informed consent and autonomy. And thank you for thinking enough of your loved ones to make their roles as decision makers—if that day ever comes—the privilege that it should be and not the burden that it could be.

Here's the practice of health literacy in a nutshell:

- Identify the issue.
- Gather information.
- Ask questions.
- Discuss your options.
- Take a deep breath.
- Make an informed decision.
- Repeat as needed.

There's heaps more I could say about health literacy, your importance as a patient and where this all may end, but we both know time is a precious commodity and I respect the value of whatever is left for you and for me.

Congratulations and welcome to the *Two Percent Club*.

GLOSSARY

Absolute risk: The odds of an event occurring, e.g., contracting a disease or being cured. *Example*: 20 percent of smokers get lung cancer.

Absolute risk reduction: The difference between the risk of occurrence in one group and the risk of the same occurrence in another group. *Example*: A nonsmoker has a 2 percent chance of getting lung cancer; compared to a smoker, that's an 18 percent absolute risk reduction.

Acute care: Medical care focused on conditions that come on suddenly and are usually of a short duration, such as appendicitis or a sprained ankle.

Advance Care Planning: Considering, communicating and documenting one's wishes for substitute decision making in the event of future incapacity and for the recognition of a proxy.

Advance Directive: see **Health Care Advance Directive**.

Artificial nutrition and hydration (tubal feeding): Liquids delivered by a tube entering the digestive system through the nose, mouth, wall of the stomach or intestine; or through an intravenous line placed into a vein for hydration and short-term nutrition.

Autonomy: Decision making incorporating the individual's personal values and moral independence, done without undue influence.

Brain death: The irreversible and permanent absence of all brain activity, including brainstem reflexes, as indicated by fixed pupils and no pain response; the patient cannot breathe without a ventilator and is considered medically dead.

Capacity (also called **decision making capacity**): The mental ability to understand the nature and consequences of an issue, make a fully informed decision regarding it and comprehend the effects of that choice.

Cardiac arrest: When a person's heart stops beating.

Cardiopulmonary resuscitation (CPR): A combination of forcing air into the lungs, compressing the chest manually or mechanically and the use of drugs and electric shock to restart the heart and maintain blood flow to the brain.

Chronic condition: A physical or mental condition that lasts a year or longer, requires ongoing medical attention and/or limits the patient's daily living activities.

Cohort: A group of persons sharing common demographic characteristics such as Baby Boomers or the Greatest Generation.

Coma: A state of deep unconsciousness from which the patient cannot be roused and there is no wakefulness or awareness. A patient may or may not awake from a coma.

Comfort Care Only: A medical order that calls for the relief of suffering without treating any underlying medical conditions or attempting emergency resuscitation.

Competency: A court's finding that a person has the ability to understand and make decisions concerning health care, everyday life and the management of assets.

Dead donor rule: The doctrine that a patient must be declared medically dead before any organs can be harvested for transplantation.

Dementia: A decline in thinking ability and memory that affects a person's ability to perform everyday activities.

Diagnosis: The identification of a disease or medical condition.

Do-not-resuscitate order (DNR): A written medical order stating that in the event a person's heart and breathing stop, resuscitation should not be attempted.

Durable Power of Attorney for Health Care: A Health Care Advance Directive in which a person delegates medical decision making authority to another person, the health care proxy, in the event of future decision making incapacity.

Emergency care: Medical treatment for a medical condition or traumatic injury that requires immediate medical attention, such as a heart attack or an automobile accident.

Endotracheal intubation: The insertion of a tube down a person's throat to provide food or water.

Ethical Will: The record of a person's beliefs and values, life lessons and hopes for the future, recorded for the benefit of loved ones or survivors.

Euthanasia: The intentional taking of a person's life by another to relieve the person's pain or suffering.

Full Code: A medical order to take all necessary measures to treat and/or revive a patient who is in a medical crisis and suffers cardiac and/or respiratory arrest.

Guardian: A court-appointed person with authority to manage the personal care of a person who lacks legal competency. (In some states, a *guardian* may also manage assets.)

Guardian ad litem: A person appointed by a court to represent the interests of a potential ward of the court under a guardianship or conservatorship during court proceedings.

Guardianship: A legal relationship giving the duty to care for a person who lacks legal competency to another, the guardian. (In some states, *guardianship* may also refer to asset management.)

Hastened death: When death occurs sooner than it would otherwise occur because of the intervention of an action.

Health Care Advance Directive: A legal document that includes a person's appointment of a substitute medical decision maker (a Durable Power of Attorney for Health Care) and directives for the use of life extending and life prolonging measures in the case of a triggering event (a Living Will). Both functions may be joined in a combination directive.

Health care proxy: A person appointed in a Health Care Advance Directive to act as a substitute decision maker for another person in the event of decision making incapacity.

Health literacy: The ability to recognize when, how and where to access, process and understand basic health information and services needed to make informed decisions in a particular health care situation.

HIPAA: The Health Insurance Portability and Accountability Act of 1996.

Hospice: An interdisciplinary approach to patient palliative care when a cure is no longer possible or a patient chooses to discontinue curative treatment, and life expectancy is six months or less. *Hospice* also refers to a residential facility for dying patients.

Hospitalist: A doctor who specializes in treating the hospitalized patients of other doctors or those without a primary care physician.

Incapacity: A lack of the mental ability to understand the nature and consequences of a situation or problem, make a decision regarding it and comprehend the effects of that choice.

Incompetency: A legal determination that a person lacks the mental ability to understand and make decisions concerning health care, everyday life or the management of assets.

Informed consent: Voluntarily agreeing to, refusing to agree to or requesting the withdrawal of a medical procedure with full understanding of the foreseeable risks, benefits, possible alternatives, uncertainties and the option of having no treatment.

Irreversible or permanent unconsciousness: A coma or vegetative state in which the patient is not aware of his surroundings and will never recover consciousness.

Intensivist: A physician who specializes in the treatment of patients in an Intensive Care Unit.

Kidney dialysis: Removing wastes and extra salt and liquids from the body by the use of mechanical means when a person's kidneys are no longer fully functioning.

Life extending measures: Medical procedures that extend a patient's life, although they do not replace a vital function, such as breathing or eating. *Example*: kidney dialysis.

Life-limiting disease: An illness that is likely to be the direct cause of a person's death sometime in the future.

Life prolonging measures: Mechanical or artificial means used to sustain a vital function, such as a ventilator for breathing or a feeding tube and IV for nutrition and hydration.

Living Will: An advance directive that specifies the patient's wishes for the use of life extending or life prolonging measures in the event of a terminal condition, irreversible unconsciousness or late stage dementia.

Malignant: A disease that is highly infectious, invasive in the human body or potentially life-threatening.

Medicaid: A joint federal and state program that provides payment for the health care of people with low income and limited resources.

Medical futility: When a medical treatment or procedure is unlikely to produce any beneficial results for the patient.

Medicare: A federal health insurance program for people aged 65 or older, younger people on Social Security disability and people with End-Stage Renal Disease.

Mobility: The measure of a person's ability to move.

Metastasis: When a cancer spreads to sites in the body not directly connected to the original site; the cancer is said to have *metastasized*; the secondary cancers are called *metastases*.

Morbidity: Disease or illness.

Mortality: Susceptibility to death, or likelihood of dying.

Nasogastric tube: A tube inserted into a person's stomach through the nasal passage.

Needs assessment: A comprehensive assessment of a person's care needs.

Out-of-hospital Do-not-resuscitate order (OOH-DNR): A portable medical order stating that resuscitation is not to be attempted if the person's breathing and heart stop outside the hospital setting.

Palliative care: A medical specialty that focuses on comfort care and quality of life by relieving the symptoms of a disease or of the side effects of medical treatment.

Palliative sedation: For pain that cannot otherwise be relieved, the use of sedative drugs to reduce the patient's level of unconsciousness.

Parenteral nutrition: The use of an intravenous line (IV) to provide nutrients to a patient.

Pharmacodynamics: The study of the effects a drug has on the body.

Pharmacokinetics: The study of how the body impacts the effects of a drug.

Physician-assisted suicide: A health care professional assists a patient to commit suicide by providing a prescription for a lethal drug to be administered by the patient.

POLST (Physician Orders for Life-Sustaining Treatment) form or **order**: A document signed by a provider and the patient (or decision maker) that turns the patient's advance directives into actionable medical orders, intended for use by terminally ill and frail patients.

Polypharmacy: The use of five or more medications by one patient.

Professional guardian: A person who is appointed by a court and paid to manage the personal care and/or the property of an incapacitated person, the ward.

Prognosis: A prediction of the probable timeline, outcome, survival rate and course of a disease or medical condition.

Provider: A health care professional who is in direct contact with the patient, such as a physician, physician's assistant, nurse practitioner, nurse, therapist, nurse's assistant, home health aide, pharmacist or staff member of a care or rehabilitation facility.

Proxy-by-statute: A person recognized by state law to make end-of-life medical and care decisions on behalf of another person who does not have a written Living Will and Durable Power of Attorney for Health Care.

Relative risk: Comparing the risk of an event occurring between two groups of people or the same group in two periods of time. *Example*: A smoker has a 20 percent chance of getting lung cancer, which is 10 times as likely as the 2 percent risk for nonsmokers.

Relative risk reduction: The reduction in risk of an event occurring, expressed as a ratio or the percentage of the decrease in risk. *Example*: Being a nonsmoker reduces your chance of getting cancer by 90 percent, compared to a smoker (20 percent vs. 2 percent).

Respiratory arrest: When a person stops breathing.

Resuscitation: See **Cardiopulmonary resuscitation (CPR)**.

Standby guardianship: Documents prepared prior to incapacity that establish a court-ordered guardianship in the event the person becomes incapacitated in the future.

Substituted judgment: When acting on behalf of a patient who lacks decision making capacity, making decisions as the patient would, if able, based on the patient's specific directives or on general or specific evidence of the patient's beliefs, values and attitudes about life.

Terminal condition: A medical condition that cannot be cured and is expected to cause the patient's death in a relatively short period of time.

Trajectory: The progression of a medical condition, from onset of the disease to the death caused by it. *Examples:* sudden death from a heart attack has a short and steep trajectory; Alzheimer's disease has a gradual and extended trajectory.

Triggering event: A medical event, such as having a terminal condition, being irreversibly unconscious or being in the final stage of dementia, that triggers the use of or withholding of life prolonging measures, as specified in the patient's directive or in a state statute.

Urgent care: Medical care for a condition or injury that requires attention as soon as possible, but is not serious enough to need the services of an emergency or trauma center.

Vegetative state: An irreversible condition as the result of brain damage, in which the patient exhibits sleep-wake cycles without any consciousness and with no cognitive function.

Ventilator: A machine that mechanically assists a patient to breathe through a tube inserted in the nose or mouth or directly into the windpipe.

Voluntary stopping of eating and drinking (VSED): The voluntary refusal of food and hydration by a patient who chooses to not prolong his life.

APPENDIX

Index of decision making dilemmas

HELP – I have some symptoms that don't seem quite right but I'm not ready to talk to my doctor about this.	Chapter **Four**
HELP – My doctor just told me I have cancer. What am I supposed to do now?	Chapters **Seven** and **Twelve**
HELP – I want to name my best friend as my health care proxy. Is that allowed and do I need to put it in writing?	Chapters **Five** and **Fifteen**
HELP – My doctor just announced his retirement. How do I find a new provider?	Chapter **Six**
HELP – I'm not sure my loved one is safe anymore at home on his own.	Chapter **Eight**
HELP – It seems like my mother gets a new prescription every time she visits a doctor. Are all those drugs really necessary?	Chapter **Ten**
HELP – I hate getting my annual checkup. Do I really need one?	Chapter **Nine**
HELP – The hospital emergency room just called—my father may have had a stroke. What should I do first?	Chapter **Eleven**
HELP – My doctor just suggested I could benefit from palliative care. I think he's trying to tell me I'm dying.	Chapter **Thirteen**
HELP – The doctor keeps suggesting more treatments for my elderly father but he's not getting any better. Is it time for hospice?	Chapters **Seven**, **Ten**, **Twelve**, **Thirteen** and **Fourteen**
HELP – Doing paperwork is boring and usually makes me feel like an idiot. Why do I need it?	Chapters **Six**, **Ten**, **Eleven** and **Fifteen**

RECOMMENDED READING

Being Mortal
Medicine and What Matters in the End
Atul Gawande

When breath becomes air
Paul Kalanithi

The Four Things That Matter Most
A Book About Living
Ira Byock, MD

tuesdays with Morrie
Mitch Albom

On Death and Dying
Elisabeth Kubler-Ross, MD

Extreme Measures
Finding a Better Path to the End of Life
Jessica Nutik Zitter, MD
(and *Extremis*, the documentary featuring
Dr. Jessica Nutik Zitter on Netflix.com)

The practical guide to
Health Care Advance Directives
Jo Kline Cebuhar, J.D.

SO GROWS THE TREE
Creating an Ethical Will
Jo Kline Cebuhar, J.D.

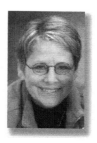

ABOUT THE AUTHOR

Attorney Jo Kline began writing about the legal and health care issues of medical decision making and end of life after her service as volunteer chair of Iowa's largest hospice. Jo's writing includes her 2015 book on Advance Care Planning, **The practical guide to Health Care Advance Directives** and the award-winning **SO GROWS THE TREE – Creating an Ethical Will**. Her first novel **EXIT**, set in a small-town hospice, was released in 2014. Jo is also the creator of a multistate Health Care Advance Directive that reflects contemporary medical conditions and treatment choices and acts as a guide for medical decision making in any health care situation.

Among other print, broadcast and online media, Jo has been featured in *The New York Times*, *Reader's Digest*, *The Philadelphia Inquirer*, *The Des Moines Register*, the *Huffington Post* and *Lifezette.com*. She is a frequent contributor to online media, a guest essayist for *The Des Moines Register* and the author of its 12-part series, "Health Literacy 101."

www.HealthLiteracy101.com

www.Advance-Directives.net

Jo's email: JoKline@msn.com

ABOUT THE COVER

The late 1800s drawing on the cover of this book depicts a chart of phrenology, which was a 19th century pseudoscience studying the shape and size of the cranium. It was believed that segments of the brain were directly linked to different emotional and intellectual functions, which could be determined by measuring the bumps and indentations in a person's skull. Except for the bumps and indentations part, they were absolutely right.

A GRAMMATICAL NOTE

I could have gone with "he" or "he or she" or "they." I went with "he." It's an editorial decision, not an ideological stance.

[1] "Hula Hoop," How Products are Made, Volume 6, www.madehow.com.

[2] Jennifer M. Ortman et al, "Aging Nation: The Older Population in the United States—Populations Estimates and Projections," May 2014, U.S. Department of Commerce, U.S. Census Bureau, www. census.gov.

[3] "Estimates of the Population of States, by Age, 1965 to 1967," Series P-25, No. 420, April 17, 1969, U.S. Department of Commerce, Bureau of the Census, www.census.gov.

[4] "Nursing Shortage Fact Sheet," April 24, 2014, American Association of Colleges of Nursing, www.aacn.nche.edu and Stephen P. Juraschek, BA et al, "United States Registered Nurse Workforce Report Card and Shortage Forecast," American Journal of Medical Quality, Volume 27, No. 3, January 2012.

[5] "National Assessment of Adult Literacy/Health Literacy," National Center for Education Statistics, U.S. Department of Education, 2003.

[6] "National Action Plan to Improve Health Literacy," U.S. Department of Health and Human Services, Office of Disease Prevention and Health Promotion, May 2010.

[7] Barry D. Weiss, M.D., "Health literacy and patient safety: Help patients understand – Manual for Clinicians (Second Edition)," 2007, American Medical Association Foundation, www.commerce.ama-assn.org.

[8] A modern parable most recently credited to the series "West Wing." Episode #32, aired December 20, 2000.

[9] Julia Quinlan interview by Barbara Manieri, Sparta Independent, January 6, 2000, www.karenannquinlanhospice.org.

[10] William H. Colby, *A Long Goodbye* (Carlsbad, California: Hay House, Inc., 2002); *Cruzan v. Director, Missouri Department of Health*, 497 U.S. 261 (1990).

[11] *In the Matter of Karen Quinlan, an Alleged Incompetent*, The Supreme Court of New Jersey, 70 N.J. 10 (1976), 355 A. 2nd 647 (1976).

[12] *In re: Guardianship of Theresa Marie Schiavo - Robert Schindler and Mary Schindler v. Michael Schiavo, as Guardian of the person of Theresa Marie Schiavo*, In the District Court of Appeal of Florida Second District, Case No. 2D02-5394, June 6, 2003 and Kathy Cerminara and Kenneth Goodman, University of Miami Ethics Programs, "Key Events in the Case of Theresa Marie Schiavo," www.miami.edu.

[13] "About the Multiple Chronic Conditions Initiative," Office of the Assistant Secretary for Health, U.S. Department of Health & Human Services, www.HHS.gov and "Chronic Condition Charts: 2015," Centers for Medicare & Medicaid Services, U.S. Department of Health & Human Services, www.cms.gov.

[14] Monroe Lerner, *When, Why and Where People Die* (New York: Russell Sage Foundation, 1970).

[15] Ferdinando L. Mirarchi, DO et al., TRIAD (The Realistic Interpretation of Advance Directives) studies, "Triad III: Nationwide Assessment of Living Wills and Do Not Resuscitate Orders," The Journal of Emergency Medicine, Volume 42, No. 5, May 2012.

[16] Susannah Fox, "The Social Life of Health Information, 2011," Pew Research Center – Internet, Science & Tech, www.pewInternet.org.

[17] Jo Kline Cebuhar, J.D., *Whose big idea was that? Lessons in giving from the pioneers of value-inspired philanthropy* (West Des Moines: Murphy Publishing, LLC, 2012). Among

others, it includes the story of Jerome Stone's relentless efforts to find answers about his wife's Alzheimer's disease, which was how the Alzheimer's Association came to be.

[18] Maria T. Carney et al, "Elder Orphans Hiding in Plain Sight: A Growing Vulnerable Population," Current Gerontology and Geriatrics Research, July 2016.

[19] *In the Matter of Karen Quinlan, an Alleged Incompetent*, The Supreme Court of New Jersey, 70 N.J. 10 (1076), 355 A. 2nd 647 (1976); "Opinion 8.081 – Surrogate Decision Making," AMA Code of Medical Ethics, American Medical Association, www.ama-assn.org.

[20] U.S. Government Information on Organ and Tissue Donation and Transplantation, U.S. Department of Health & Human Services, "State Organ Donation Legislation," www.organdonor.gov/legislation_micro.

[21] The President's Commission for the Study of Ethical Problems in Medicine and Biomedical and Behavioral Research, U.S. Government Printing Office, Washington, D.C., 1982.

[22] Agency for Healthcare Research and Quality, "The SHARE Approach—Essential Steps of Shared Decisionmaking: Expanded Reference Guide with Sample Conversation Starters," U.S. Department of Health and Human Services, www.ahrq.gov.

[23] Drawing on all of the following sources: Jo Kline Cebuhar, J.D., *The practical guide to Health Care Advance Directives*, (West Des Moines: Murphy Publishing, LLC, 2015); Atul Gawande, *Being Mortal – Medicine and What Matters in the End* (New York: Metropolitan Books – Henry Holt and Company, LLC, 2014); Ezekiel J. Emanuel and Linda L. Emanuel, "Four models of the physician-patient relationship," The Journal of the American Medical Association, Volume 267, Number 16, April 22, 1992; and "The SHARE Approach—Essential Steps of Shared Decisionmaking: Expanded Reference Guide With Sample Conversations Starters," Agency for Healthcare Research and Quality, www.ahrz.gov.

[24] "Caregiving in the U.S. 2009," National Alliance for Caregiving in Collaboration with AARP, 2009, www.caregiving.org.

[25] Donald Redfoot et al, "The Aging of the Baby Boom and the Growing Care Gap: A Look at Future Declines in the Availability of Family Caregivers," Insight on the Issues, AARP Public Policy Institute, August 2013.

[26] "Kaiser Health Tracking Poll: November, 2014," the Henry J. Kaiser Family Foundation, www.kff.org.

[27] "National Action Plan to Improve Health Literacy," U.S. Department of Health and Human Services, Office of Disease Prevention and Health Promotion, May 2010.

[28] "Total number of retail prescription drugs filled at pharmacies (2016)," Henry J. Kaiser Family Foundation, www.kff.org.

[29] "Taking medicines – what to ask your doctor," MedlinePlus, National Institutes of Health, U.S. National Library of Medicine, www.https://medlineplus.gov.

[30] "ASCP Fact Sheet," American Society of Consultant Pharmacists, www.ASCP.com.

[31] Ferdinando Mirarchi, DO, FAAEM, FACEP, "A New Nationwide Patient Safety Concern Related to Living Wills, DNR Orders, and POLST-Like Documents," National Patient Safety Foundation, "Patient Safety Blog," www.npsf.org; Robert Glatter, MD and Ferdinando L. Mirarchi, DO, "Advance Directives May Be Hazardous to Your Health," Medscape Internal Medicine, www.medscape.com.

[32] "Absolute Risk and Relative Risk," Patient, www.patient.info.

[33] Naveen Sulakshan Salins et al, "Integration of Early Specialist Palliative Care in Cancer Care and Patient Related Outcomes: A Critical Review of Evidence," Indian Journal of Palliative Care, Volume 22, No. 3, July-September 2016.

[34] Jennifer S. Temel, M.D. et al, "Early Palliative Care for Patients with Metastatic Non-Small-Cell Lung Cancer," The New England Journal of Medicine, Volume 363, No. 8, August 19, 2010.

[35] Atul Gawande, "Atul Gawande: The Problem of Hubris," BBC Radio 4 Reith Lectures, World Society of Edinburgh, December 9, 2014, www.bbc.co.uk.

[36] Paul Kalanithi, *When Breath Becomes Air* (New York: Random House, 2016).

[37] "End of Life Care, Inpatient days per decedent during the last six months of life, by gender and level of care intensity: Year 2012," The Dartmouth Atlas of Health Care, www.dartmouthatlas.org.

[38] Centers for Disease Control and Prevention, National Center for Health Statistics, Health, United States, 2010: With Special Feature on Death and Dying, Data table for Figure 33. Place of death, over time: United States, 1989, 1997 and 2007, www.cdc.gov/nchs.

[39] Margaret Jean Hall, PhD et al., "Trends in Inpatient Hospital Deaths: National Hospital Discharge Survey, 2000-2010," U.S. Department of Health and Human Services, March 2013, www.cdc.gov/nchs.

[40] "NHPCO Facts and Figures – Hospice Care in America," 2015 Edition, National Hospice and Palliative Care Organization, www.NHPCO.org.

[41] Jo Kline Cebuhar, J.D., *SO GROWS THE TREE – Creating an Ethical Will* (West Des Moines: Murphy Publishing, LLC, 2010).